Chronic Fat

Megan Arroll holds a PhD in psych
and a chartered scientist. She has
ically unexplained and misundersto   .... and has
published numerous academic papers on the topic of chronic fatigue
syndrome/myalgic encephalomyelitis (CFS/ME). Megan is a member of
Action for ME's Research Panel and an expert patient representative on
the UK ME/CFS Biobank steering group. She has a close working part-
nership with Professor Christine Dancey, with whom she recently wrote
Invisible Illnesses: Coping with misunderstood conditions, also published by
Sheldon Press. Megan and Christine are both members of the Chronic
Illness Research Team based at the University of East London.

Overcoming Common Problems Series

Selected titles

A full list of titles is available from Sheldon Press,
36 Causton Street, London SW1P 4ST and on our website at
www.sheldonpress.co.uk

Overcoming Common Problems Series

Overcoming Common Problems Series

Overcoming Common Problems

Chronic Fatigue Syndrome
What you need to know about CFS/ME

DR MEGAN A. ARROLL

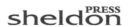

First published in Great Britain in 2014

Sheldon Press
36 Causton Street
London SW1P 4ST
www.sheldonpress.co.uk

The author and publisher have made every effort to ensure that the external
website and email addresses included in this book are correct and up to date at the
time of going to press. The author and publisher are not responsible for the content,
quality or continuing accessibility of the sites.

British Library Cataloguing-in-Publication Data
A catalogue record for this book is available from the British Library

ISBN 978–1–84709–300–4
eBook ISBN 978–1–84709–301–1

Typeset by Caroline Waldron, Wirral, Cheshire
First printed in Great Britain by Ashford Colour Press
Subsequently digitally reprinted in Great Britain

eBook by Fakenham Prepress Solutions, Fakenham, Norfolk NR21 8NN

Produced on paper from sustainable forests

I'd like to dedicate this book to my Ma. I can't imagine how hard it must have been in those first few years when I was so very ill. You are the strongest – and most talented – woman I know and I love you more than anything. We did it, you and me; we really did. Thank you.

Contents

Foreword

No other illness is surrounded by the uncertainty and sometimes profound differences of medical opinion that affect people with chronic fatigue syndrome/myalgic encephalomyelitis (CFS/ME).

With no clear agreement on what causes CFS/ME, what it should be called and how it should be diagnosed and managed, this is clearly a very challenging condition for doctors.

At the same time it can be a very frustrating medical journey for patients when it comes to obtaining a diagnosis, receiving appropriate advice on management and knowing what to do about all the other ways CFS/ME affects normal daily life.

Not surprisingly, many people disengage from conventional medicine and end up becoming expert patients in the self-management of CFS/ME.

In this book, Megan Arroll brings together her personal experience of CFS/ME, her extensive professional involvement of researching the condition, and carefully dissects the debate into the roles of the biological, psychological and social factors.

Despite all these uncertainties, Megan succeeds in bringing together what we so far know about CFS/ME in a way that is logical and easy to understand for people with no medical background.

She then translates this information into extremely helpful practical guidance on how to manage all the key symptoms – fatigue, brain fog, sleep disturbance – along with how to deal with all the problems that occur when living with CFS/ME.

As a doctor who also has CFS/ME, I found Megan's book to be full of sensible, practical and thought-provoking information.

Above all it will form a very useful source of reference for anyone who wants to become an expert patient!

Dr Charles Shepherd,
Medical Advisor to the ME Association

Preface

Chronic fatigue syndrome – these three words sound so simple and innocuous, but as I know from personal experience, when put together like this they stand for an illness that is neither simple nor trivial. I was diagnosed with CFS/ME when I was 14, after a bout of glandular fever (though the process of gaining a diagnosis was also not at all straightforward), and at that time I was completely awash with what felt like hundreds of different symptoms. I felt confused and utterly overwhelmed; a feeling that I again experienced when I started my PhD on the topic some eight years later. I thought there couldn't be very much research in the area as no one yet had any definitive answers as to the cause of the condition. I was very wrong indeed. There are a vast number of research studies and papers on the topic but, like the condition, much of the evidence is seemingly con-tradictory. I have spent my research career since – a further ten years – trying to make sense of all of this information and also adding to the evidence with my own work. This will of course change when new research is funded and published, and I'm quite sure that in the next ten years there will be even more clues to the underlying nature of the condition and additional treatment options for people with CFS/ME.

There are different ways to read this book, depending on where you are with your illness. If you simply want to know about treatments and things you can do to improve your symptoms, please skip to Chapters 6–9. Then, when you are feeling less fatigued and symptomatic, you might be interested to learn about the history of the condition and the current understanding of CFS/ME, which can be found in Chapters 1 and 2. Further theories about the development and perpetuation of CFS/ME are outlined in Chapters 3 and 4. It must be stated, however, that this is not an exhaustive discussion of the models of CFS/ME – there are quite a few out there and it would be beyond the scope of this book to include every theory. Chapter 5 talks a bit more about symptoms, while the final chapter, Chapter 10, presents the very encouraging progress that has been made in recent years within the research and medical CFS/ME world. Finally, it is worth noting that the material for this book draws on both current research and practice and real-life experiences of people with CFS/ME. I do hope you find it useful and informative.

Acknowledgements

A heartfelt thanks go to my buddy Christine Dancey. Apart from the practical help you've given me in terms of reviewing drafts and proof-reading, the support you've so generously provided at every stage of this book and our other projects has been invaluable. It has also made 'work' a great deal of fun!

I'd also like to thank Jo Johnstone, who has taught me a few things about English grammar that I didn't know – thank you. The time you've spent reading and proof-reading is totally and completely appreciated.

Thanks to Charles Shepherd for writing the Foreword to this book. Charles has been both an inspiration and a huge support to me over the years. I look forward to seeing what the future holds for this condition with you, Charles. I'd also like to thank Carolyn Appleby for her wise advice.

Finally but not by any means least importantly I would like to thank everyone who has participated in my research over the years and provided the material for the case studies in this book (naturally names have been changed for this purpose). Your participation is the only way we will continue to gain understanding of not just CFS/ME but also other complex illnesses.

Note to the reader

This is not a medical book and is not intended to replace advice from your doctor. Consult your pharmacist or doctor if you believe you have any of the symptoms described, and if you think you might need medical help.

1

Chronic fatigue syndrome: what's in a name?

The wisdom of naming a disorder, the nature of which cannot at present be proved, and which may be due to more than one agent, is debatable. (Sir Ernest Donald Acheson)

In this first chapter we will take an abridged tour of the history of chronic fatigue syndrome/myalgic encaphalomyelitis (CFS/ME). As you can imagine, an entire book could be written about this, so we will just look at some of the events that influenced the naming of the disorder to try to understand not only how we ended up with the label CFS/ME but also to appreciate that it is not by any means a new condition.

If CFS/ME is not a new condition, has it been called something else in the past? If we look back in time it seems that CFS/ME has been documented as far back in history as the mid-1800s, when there was evidence of an illness that caused fatigue, pain and other symptoms associated with severe exhaustion; this condition was known as 'neurasthenia'. This term was coined by the American neurologist George Miller Beard in 1869. Beard saw neurasthenia as an illness where people pushed themselves beyond their physical and mental limits in the burgeoning new world, resulting in total exhaustion of the central nervous system. However, Beard did not believe this to be a long-term illness, perhaps because at the time people were advised to rest and convalesce in order to recover and so the symptoms didn't turn into a long-term condition.

Myalgic encephalomyelitis

Let's now fast-forward to the mid-1900s. In 1955, at the infectious disease clinic within the Royal Free Hospital in north London, a number of patients were admitted with a viral-like illness. In the beginning the symptoms seemed quite ordinary – sore throat, slight fever and so on – but then something very strange seemed to happen. A raft of new symptoms started to be reported by the patients, including headaches, problems with memory and concentration and, perhaps most notably, extreme muscle fatigue following the smallest amount of exercise. The doctors could not put their finger on the cause of the illness as some of the symptoms suggested polio but other classic features of the disease – such as muscle wastage – were not found. Some, but not all, patients had abnormal brain activity as demonstrated by electroencephalogram (EEG) results, which led to the conclusion that they were experiencing brain inflammation or 'encephalitis'.

Then later that same year, 292 people became ill at the hospital with a flu-like illness. The striking thing about this apparent outbreak was that of the 292 cases, only 12 were patients – the rest were hospital staff, mostly doctors and nurses. As so many staff were now ill, the hospital was forced to close, making this outbreak quite famous at the time. In 1956 a leading article published in *The Lancet* suggested that this illness be understood as 'a new clinical entity' and named 'benign myalgic encephalomyelitis'. This name was suggested because some of the symptoms of people in the Royal Free outbreak seemed to involve inflammation of the nervous system (problems with how messages were transmitted from the brain to the muscles via nerves), hence the medical term 'myelitis'. In addition there was also the severe muscle pain and tenderness or 'myalgia'. Therefore this name represents:

benign – people did not die from this illness, although they could certainly be very unwell
myalgic – severe muscle pain
encephalo – disease of the brain
myelitis – inflammation of the nervous system

The term 'myalgic encephalomyelitis' or 'ME' is commonly used now, especially by charities (Action for ME, the ME Association, ME Research UK). However, there has been much debate about whether this is the correct name for the illness. In 1959, following the outbreak at the Royal Free Hospital and after 14 additional similar outbreaks in Iceland, Australia, Europe, the USA and South Africa, Sir Ernest Donald Acheson investigated the characteristics of these illnesses. Acheson, who died in 2010, was an eminent British doctor and epidemiologist (that is, someone who studies the frequency and distribution of diseases), and was Chief Medical Officer for the Department of Health from 1983 to 1991. In his review he found that more than

1,000 people were affected in these 14 outbreaks, and notably in seven of the outbreaks many nurses and doctors had fallen ill, just as at the Royal Free. The aim of this task was to see if these outbreaks that had been reported all over the world were indeed one and the same illness. This was a tricky exercise, as Sir Donald pointed out:

> The difficulties in defining a disorder from which no deaths have occurred, and for which no causative infective or toxic agent has been discovered, are obvious. Recognition has to depend on the clinical and epidemiology pattern. These features must be sufficiently characteristic to separate the disorder from other conditions.

He stated that all the outbreaks shared the following characteristics:

- headache;
- myalgia;
- muscular paresis (or weakness);
- symptoms or signs other than paresis suggestive of damage to the brain, spinal cord or peripheral nerves;
- mental symptoms;
- low or absent fever in most cases;
- no mortality.

Also, more women than men had succumbed to the illnesses, the patients had predominantly normal cerebrospinal fluid, relapses occurred in almost all the outbreaks and all age groups – from late childhood to people in their eighties – were affected. But what was very striking was the proportion of medical staff who became ill: in the outbreak in Florida, 40 per cent of medical personnel had symptoms of this strange illness. The illness did not seem to be spread by food or water, rather by person-to-person contact. However, in all the medical tests that were carried out – for instance blood test, tests to look for bacterial causes, EEGs – there was no clear, identifiable cause that could be seen. But because there were indeed so many similarities in terms of the symptoms and the way the illness affected people, Acheson was able to conclude: 'The disease is recognizable in its epidemic form on clinical and epidemiologic grounds and therefore may properly be considered a clinical entity.'

Because an exact cause could not be found, Acheson suggested that the term 'benign myalgic encephalomyelitis' be used until new and more conclusive evidence should come to light, and he quoted Jean-Martin Charcot (1825–93), a French neurologist sometimes referred to as 'the father of neurology', to emphasize this point: 'Disease is very old and nothing about it has changed. It is we who change as we learn to recognize what was formerly imperceptible.'

Mass hysteria

This is, of course, not the end of the story. During the 1960s the name of this condition was still in question and the new evidence that Acheson had hoped for had yet to emerge. Then, in 1970, two British psychiatrists, Colin McEvedy and A. W. Beard, re-analysed the clinical notes from the Royal Free Hospital outbreak and concluded in a paper published in the *British Medical Journal* that 'there is little evidence of an organic disease affecting the central nervous system and that epidemic hysteria is a much more likely explanation'. McEvedy and Beard based these conclusions on the facts that: more women than men had become ill; the 'malaise' or fatigue was severe even though fevers tended to be mild; there was a lack of positive blood and other laboratory tests. They compared the cases at the Royal Free to those of an epidemic of overbreathing in schoolgirls, which McEvedy had studied a few years earlier. It was pointed out that the two epidemics shared common features, such as feeling hot and cold, perceptual problems, disorientation, pins and needles and bladder dysfunction. The two psychiatrists also went on to look at the 14 outbreaks Acheson had studied and an additional one that had occurred after his review, and stated:

> We believe that a lot of these epidemics were psychosocial phenomena caused by one of two mechanisms, either mass hysteria on the part of the patients or altered medical perception of the community. We suggest that the name 'myalgia nervosa' should be used for any future cases of functional disorder which present the same clinical picture.

This was very much at odds with Acheson's statement that 'no one can seriously contend that every patient in all the outbreaks described in this paper has been hysterical'. These opposing opinions led to a great deal of debate about whether this illness was physical in nature (due to a viral infection) or psychiatric (mass hysteria).

Chronic Epstein-Barr syndrome

During the 1970s and 1980s there were more epidemics, most famously that of 1984 in Lake Tahoe in the USA. This quite exclusive destination was popular with the affluent professionals at the time, the high achievers of the 1980s who worked hard and were handsomely rewarded for their efforts – that is, not people seemingly likely to take time off sick.

> I'd read a headline in the newspaper, something about yuppie flu, and I remember thinking as I read it: 'I don't even have time to read that article. Those yuppies – I don't know what's wrong with them! Boy am I ill! They should know what illness is like!' I didn't realize it was the same illness that we all had. (Mary)

Like Mary, many people doubted whether the group of high-flying professionals had a genuine illness. This may be because it wasn't easy for many people to identify with the condition from media descriptions, while the medics continued to report that all the tests were coming back negative and/or inconclusive. Therefore there was still a great deal of uncertainty as to what the condition actually *was*, and what it *was not*. Doctors and scientists started to wonder if the outbreaks were due to glandular fever (known in the USA as infectious mononucleosis), which is caused by a virus called the Epstein-Barr virus (EBV). The symptoms of EBV are very similar to those reported in the epidemics: sore throats, raised temperature, body and headaches and, most tellingly, swollen glands. In some cases the name 'chronic Epstein-Barr syndrome' was used, which added yet another name to the mix. But there was a problem with this theory: EBV is a herpesvirus, like cold sores, chicken pox and genital herpes, and by adulthood the vast majority of the population have antibodies to it, which means they should be immune to it. However, herpesviruses can lie dormant in the body and later become reactivated; for instance, shingles is a reactivation of chicken pox later in life, usually caused by a strain on the immune system triggered possibly by older age or high levels of stress. If you are someone who is prone to cold sores, you might have also noticed that they appear during stressful times.

Two doctors, Dan Peterson and Paul Cheney, wanted to see if this is what had happened to the people at Lake Tahoe, so they collected blood samples and checked them for active EBV. At first the findings seemed promising, about three quarters of the group showing positive results, but in the end the proportion of those with active EBV was about the same as the general population. So it seemed that the label 'chronic Epstein-Barr syndrome' wasn't accurate after all.

At the time of writing, Paul Cheney still conducts research into CFS/ME and runs a CFS/ME clinic in Ashville, North Carolina. Dan Peterson has also dedicated his career to the study and treatment of CFS/ME and was part of the panel who devised the Fukuda criteria, the most commonly used guidelines (see Chapter 2). In 2005 he helped set up the Whittemore Peterson Institute for Neuro-Immune Diseases in Nevada, which studies CFS/ME and related disorders. Hence these doctors certainly believe there are underlying physiological issues in CFS/ME, but at the time of the Lake Tahoe outbreak EBV didn't appear to be the answer.

Post-viral fatigue syndrome

> I'd actually seen my own GP, who said: 'You've got post-viral . . .' What's it called? Post-viral syndrome. I'd never heard of that. I remember at one point saying: 'What happens if the virus doesn't get better?' He said: 'Oh, you don't get viruses like that'! (Caroline)

This search for a virus had sparked some interest though. Because it was the 1980s and the HIV/AIDS epidemic was spreading fast and devastating lives, viruses were getting a lot of attention from scientists, funding bodies and the press. Dr David Bell, who like Peterson and Cheney studied an outbreak (this time in Lyndonville, a town in a rural area of the state of New York), also felt that the condition was caused by a viral infection, and in 1987 he joined a group of researchers interested in retroviruses. In 1991 the group published findings that linked CFS/ME to the human T-lymphotropic viruses 1 and 2 (known as HTLV1 and HTLV2), which are retroviruses. However, consensus was still not reached: different studies often found different culprits. David Bell spent many years treating those with CFS/ME and carrying out research. He is now retired but has conducted a 13-year follow-up of the children in the Lyndonville outbreak, published in 2001, which found that 80 per cent of the children had recovered or adapted to a satisfactory degree.

Chronic fatigue syndrome

As you can see, the picture was becoming more rather than less confusing, the more research was done. There were also names such as 'chronic fatigue immune deficiency syndrome' (CFIDS), which is still used in the USA due to the support group CFIDS Association. All these different labels were causing a great deal of confusion and it was hard to tell if they related to one and the same condition or many different ones – the results of research studies were often inconclusive or the findings could not be replicated. Therefore in 1988 a group of expert scientists and doctors met to discuss just that: Was this one or many illnesses? This was organized by the national Centers for Disease Control and Prevention, a prominent health organization based in Atlanta, Georgia and led by Dr Gary Holmes, a specialist in internal medicine and infectious disease, with special expertise in CFS/ME and herpes infections. The group reviewed the published evidence in order to agree a 'case definition' – a set of criteria that defines a condition. As they could not see enough evidence for EBV or any of the other viruses, the group settled on the term 'chronic fatigue syndrome'. This new label reflected the main, outwardly clinical characteristic without alluding to an underlying physical cause and, hence, the definition was based on signs and symptoms rather than diagnostic tests. This was the basis for the Fukuda case definition, which we will discuss in Chapter 2.

In 1992 chronic fatigue syndrome entered the World Health Organization's International Statistical Classification of Diseases and Related Health Problems as an alternative term for post-viral fatigue syndrome and benign myalgic encephalomyelitis. However, many people use the term ME/CFS or CFS/ME as it is felt that CFS may trivialize a severe and debilitating condition. Therefore in this book we will use the abbreviation CFS/ME. Until we know the exact cause and nature of the disorder, as Sir Ernest Donald Acheson stated in the quote above, none of these labels will be satisfactory.

Summary and conclusion

In this chapter we have explored the way CFS/ME has been named over time and also highlighted where some of the confusion about the disorder may have originated. Now that we know a bit about the history of CFS/ME, we can proceed to see what is happening currently in theory and treatment and also look towards the future.

2

So what exactly is chronic fatigue syndrome?

Moving along from the history of CFS/ME, we will now look at the current definitions of CFS/ME and then explore how the condition impacts people's lives. You may see some of your experiences mirrored in the description of the condition in the case studies drawn from others with CFS/ME, which may be upsetting. Please remember that gaining knowledge of an illness is an important part of dealing with it and taking back a sense of control. In later chapters we will outline different ways you can start to regain your health, including techniques you can practise at home by yourself and approaches you may want to explore with healthcare practitioners – doctors, psychologists, nurses and so on.

So to start to unpick the term chronic fatigue syndrome, as we discussed what ME means in the previous chapter, let's first look at the words that make up the name:

chronic – long lasting, as opposed to an acute condition, such as appendicitis, which can be dealt with and the patient will be 'cured';
fatigue – tiredness, 'malaise', lack of energy and so on;
syndrome – a collection of symptoms; used to label an illness when no one is sure of its 'aetiology' or cause.

If you're looking at this explanation and thinking; 'That definition doesn't cover the half of what's going on with me!', then I would agree. It does not. In fact just the symptom of 'fatigue' can mean so many different things and get confused with everyday tiredness; also there are different types of fatigue, which we will explore in Chapter 5. But let's start by looking at the current case definitions of CFS/ME, which have been extended on from the original criteria outlined in Chapter 1.

Current CFS/ME case definitions

All conditions have a case definition, which is a detailed explanation and list of symptoms that define the illness. These are devised by panels of doctors and researchers seen as experts in the field. From time to time they will form a group and get together and agree the case definition for specific conditions; this is especially important in illnesses defined by a collection of symptoms rather than an organic cause, such as a tumour. So a case definition gives the criteria for the illness – the set of symptoms a person would need to experience to be diagnosed with it. The most commonly used criteria in CFS/ME were constructed by a group of scientists and medics in 1994, also at the Centers for Disease Control and Prevention in Atlanta. This group was led by Dr Keiji Fukuda, an expert in infectious disease – most notably influenza – and now the Assistant Director-General for Health Security and Environment at the World Health Organization. The group studied the first definition of CFS/ME (which we looked at in Chapter 1), the available published research and also took into account the clinical experiences of the medics in the group. The case definition of 1988 was updated, and how it stands at present is as follows (known as the 'Fukuda guidelines').

The main symptom is fatigue; this fatigue needs to be persistent (constant) or relapsing (comes and goes, perhaps with activity), and needs to be present for at least six months. Also, the fatigue must have just started (that is, to meet the criterion for the symptom of 'fatigue', you couldn't have been experiencing it for years), or it needs to be very obvious when it started (that is, 'of definite onset'). Any other conditions that may cause this fatigue must be ruled out before a diagnosis of CFS/ME is made, for instance thyroid problems, diagnosable sleep conditions, major depression, anorexia and bulimia nervosa, obesity, side effects from various drugs (the list is quite extensive). Once all these other possible causes are ruled out, then – and only then – would it be possible to diagnose CFS/ME based on the following symptoms (at least four need to be present to meet the case criteria):

1 cognitive impairment – that is, difficulties in memory and/or concentration;
2 sore throat;
3 tender lymph nodes in the neck or armpit;
4 muscle pain;
5 multi-joint pain;

6 headaches (of a new type, pattern or severity at onset);
7 unrefreshing sleep;
8 post-exertion malaise – that is, extreme tiredness that lasts more than 24 hours after activity.

This may start to sound a little bit more like what you've experienced, but you may think it doesn't cover everything that's been going on in your body. Another group of experts agreed that this definition missed out a lot of what people with CFS/ME were experiencing. In 2003 they met and created a new set of criteria. They were led by Dr Bruce Carruthers, a specialist in internal medicine from Canada, who himself has treated many hundreds of patients with CFS/ME. This working group developed a much more comprehensive set of criteria, and this new case definition – the 'Canadian criteria' – is increasingly being used in research studies. In addition to excluding any other fatiguing conditions, you must experience fatigue that limits daily activity (that is, it is hard to carry out household chores that would previously have been done quite easily), the 'post-exertional malaise', unrefreshing sleep, pain (muscles/joint pain and/or headaches) and cognitive problems (two or more from a long list that includes sensitivity to light and noise). But in addition to these, an individual must also have at least one symptom from two of the following three categories:

1 Autonomic manifestations – for example, very pale skin, light-headedness, urinary frequency. These stem from the autonomic nervous system, which is part of the nervous system that controls bodily functions such as heart and respiratory rates, digestion, urination and pupil dilation.
2 Neuroendocrine manifestations – for example, sweating episodes, intolerance of heat and cold, marked weight change or abnormal appetite. The neuroendocrine system refers to the combined nervous and endocrine systems, which interact and regulate numerous processes within the body. For instance, the neuroendocrine system is important in mood regulation, blood pressure and how energy is utilized in the body (metabolism).
3 Immune manifestations – for example, recurrent sore throat, recurrent flu-like symptoms, new sensitivities to food, medications or chemicals. The immune system acts to protect the body from infections and disease. It comprises a range of defence mechanisms that normally differentiate between foreign invaders such as viruses and bacteria, and our own cells and tissues. However, sometimes our

bodies mistakenly initiate an immune response against our own bodily substances and tissues, which results in autoimmune diseases such as Addison's disease, coeliac disease and Cushing's syndrome.

This new definition also stated that the onset of CFS/ME may be gradual, which is a criterion that previously would have been excluded in the Fukuda guidelines. Also, the time from the start of symptoms to diagnosis was shortened for children from six to three months because the group recognized the importance of early diagnosis for recovery.

So we can see that certainly CFS/ME is not just about fatigue, although this can be the most debilitating symptom for some people. But regardless of which symptoms you have and to what degree, CFS/ME undoubtedly impacts on life – a topic we will now explore.

A confusing mess of symptoms

As mentioned above, CFS/ME is a syndrome, which is a collection of symptoms. These can often seem confusing: it isn't always clear how they fit together (we'll look at some of the theories as to why there is so much variation in symptoms in Chapters 3 and 4), which at times can feel overwhelming, as Deborah points out.

> I couldn't actually explain, of course, how many things were going wrong all at the same time, so for me it was just a wilderness and I was completely drowning in symptoms. (Deborah)

This sense of confusion can be quite frightening, but be assured: it is not at all unusual in CFS/ME, and with support, either from this book, your doctor or a CFS/ME support group (or all three), you can begin to make sense of what is going on in your body and mind. Another thing that can make it difficult to know whether you have CFS/ME or not is the fact that the condition has many of the same symptoms as others; indeed most long-term conditions have a fatigue component, which is why it is important to make sure you don't have another condition with a clear underlying cause that could be treated (such as a treatable sleep disorder). In fact many people only come to realize they may have CFS/ME after a friend or a colleague mentions it to them, as Lucy describes.

> One of the women I was at college with was very concerned that I wasn't well. I was in my third year and we'd got quite friendly, and it was her who said to me: 'I think you've got ME.' My husband was away for a weekend, and when he came back he'd been in a bookshop and

tossed a book over to me and said: 'This is what you've got,' and it was a book about ME. I mean, he'd read through it and he'd said: 'That's you.' So then I started reading a bit more about it, and I think I got in touch with the ME Association and what have you. That was when I thought: 'Yes, this is ME.' (Lucy)

Perhaps you had a similar experience to Lucy and this is why you're reading this book. By the time you've finished reading it, I hope you will have more understanding of CFS/ME and also the options available to improve your health.

Illness intrusiveness and impact on life

'Illness intrusiveness' is a topic my colleagues and I have studied, not only in CFS/ME but also other conditions, such as Ménière's disease – an inner-ear disorder that can cause balance problems, vertigo and tinnitus. It has also been looked at by other researchers in illnesses where the exact cause is known, such as HIV and lung cancer. The concept of illness intrusiveness relates to the degree to which an illness affects everyday life. Numerous areas of life are included – for instance, health, diet, work, personal finance, relationship with your partner, sex life, relationships with family members, active recreation (such as sports like football and tennis), passive recreation (such as reading or watching a movie) and self-expression/self-improvement, among others. The concept of illness intrusiveness is not only important to measure the impact an illness has on someone's life but also because until aspects of life are scuppered, you may not be aware that there is a health issue at the heart of some 'everyday' symptoms such as tiredness, as Peter points out:

I'm sure I had the symptoms for other things beforehand but I didn't actually think about it because although it did incapacitate me to a certain extent, I was still able to do things. I was able to work and able to get out and about. People don't always concentrate on the fact that they're ill. I never used to think in terms of being ill; it was just some sort of weakness from getting a bit older, and you don't realize that actually you are ill. (Peter)

However, in research studies, people who have CFS/ME generally report higher levels of illness intrusiveness than even those with conditions that may engender stigma (such as HIV and lung cancer) and also conditions similar to CFS/ME (such as irritable bowel syndrome (IBS)) that do not have a known cause. This may be because of the unpredictable nature of CFS/ME – people can start to feel better and then, seemingly out of nowhere, symptoms start up again (we'll look in Chapter 7 at how to prevent this pattern occurring). As Mary says, symptoms can fluctuate day-to-day, week-to-week, even month-to-month:

> I did have periods of relapse and remission, periods – maybe six weeks – where I'd be really bad or couldn't even tell anyone because I was too ill to pay attention, and then at a certain hour of a certain day I would just get a bit better and I'd be middling for a while, a few more weeks – and then it would start all over again and I was just never able to make rhyme or reason of what caused it. (Mary)

This varying illness course can make it very difficult to make plans. People with CFS/ME often feel incredibly guilty about having to break plans and engagements, as Anna says:

> I feel very guilty about it. I think that is the big thing with ME – I feel like I let people down and I've got this thing: I hate letting people down. (Anna)

Guilt can also come about from not being able, or finding it hard, to maintain 'roles' – as a mother, husband, friend, colleague and so on.

> My daughter knows about it and she's very sweet. 'It's not your fault Mummy, you're tired,' she says. I have guilt with that, because sometimes I feel I could do more. I could be a better mother if I had more energy. (Anna)

However, do remember that having an illness is not your 'fault'; right now, you need to show yourself the compassion and understanding you would show others. This can be very difficult for people who give a lot to others, and unfortunately 'givers' and 'care-takers' are often the ones who become unwell with CFS/ME (we'll look at why this is in Chapters 3 and 4). Just because CFS/ME is not a 'visible' illness, it does not make it less real for you or anyone else who has these types of conditions – others include IBS, fibromyalgia, migraine and mal de débarquement syndrome.

Fluctuating symptoms and unpredictability

The picture of why CFS/ME may be more intrusive than other illnesses becomes clearer when we take into account the fluctuations in symptoms. This can affect many areas of life but especially the fun parts such as hobbies – both active and passive recreation – as these can be the first things we lose when our health deteriorates. As we all need a roof over our heads and food to eat, the small amounts of energy those with CFS/ME have are usually used to maintain jobs and childcare. Peter tells us how he excluded almost all areas of life to work and study at the same time as having CFS/ME:

> Well, I really came unstuck with this studying and working – it nearly killed me, not literally, but my life for those three years was going to college in the evenings and working all through the day. It was pretty miserable; I had very little social life and so that's why I took that year off to do that final part. I decided I would work a 30-hour week: I would study six hours a day – three hours in the morning, three in the after- noon – week in, week out, and I would have the weekends off. (Peter)

This pressure in itself can then bring about worry, anxiety and even feelings of depression; as Peter says, 'It was pretty miserable.' These feelings are completely understandable, but this is not to say that anxiety and depression *cause* CFS/ME; however, there is a physiologic- al relationship between psychological distress and ill health, which we will look at in Chapter 4.

But for many people CFS/ME does also impact on working life, and this has further implications, as Mandy states:

> I can't work full-time, that's the biggest difference. I mean that just impacts on everything really – money, social life, purpose in life, getting by in this society. (Mandy)

In 2005 researchers within the Department of Occupational Therapy at the University of Illinois in Chicago reviewed the range of scientific literature and found that (depending on the study) anywhere between 26 and 89 per cent of people had lost their jobs because of the symp- toms of CFS/ME. Unemployment rates in those with CFS/ME varied between 35 per cent and 69 per cent of people in the studies. The reasons for these job losses and unemployment rates were numerous and included difficulties with getting up in the morning (perhaps due to fatigue) and inability to get to work (most people find commuting exhausting, so this is perhaps not surprising). When at work, people found it hard to communicate effectively, had difficulties with cogni- tive tasks and concentration, which sometimes led to errors, actually falling asleep at work and also a heightened reliance on co-workers, as Mary mentions:

I just couldn't do anything with the same strength that I used to be able to. I was still trying to be at work and I began doing things I'd never done before in the NHS, like trying to get other people to do things for me: 'Would you just run to X-rays' – while I sat on my bum because I just didn't have the energy to do it. At the hospital they could tell something was wrong with me; I don't know what they thought. I also couldn't remember things, which was very embarrassing. They invited me to change my job to a less responsible one, so instead of being in charge of a whole ward I was put in out-patients and opted to work part-time. That was easier, and I carried on like that a bit longer until I got referred to a consultant, who then in turn diagnosed my illness and wrote me off work, bless him. And I've never been back. (Mary)

This is not to say there is no hope for people with CFS/ME. There is an increasing understanding of this illness, which has led, and is leading to, even more new treatments and techniques you can try for yourself (see Chapters 6–10). But it is important to know that if you are having problems at work, in your relationships or have had to give up some activities you previously enjoyed, you are not alone and it is not because you are not trying. In fact the opposite may be true: you may be trying far too hard when your body needs some time to recover.

CFS/ME and other disorders

CFS/ME is very similar to other disorders such as fibromyalgia syndrome, IBS and multiple chemical sensitivity. Indeed many people have more than one of these conditions. Some scientists and researchers even feel that all these conditions should be lumped into one category of 'functional somatic syndromes'. This term simply means illnesses that lead a person to suffer with various symptoms, but for which there is no clear biomedical cause. The alternative view is that these are distinct illnesses, and lumping them together only makes research more difficult. However, in terms of treatment many of the options available are very similar for all of these conditions.

Although CFS/ME should not be confused with depression, a large proportion of people with CFS/ME can also have the symptoms of depression. In the past some researchers thought CFS/ME was caused by depression. Now it seems clear that having CFS/ME, a debilitating and confusing illness, can lead people to feel depressed – that is, the symptoms of depression may be a consequence of CFS/ME rather than its cause.

Summary and conclusion

Having to give up work, not being able to see friends and having difficulties with partners can all lead to a sense of isolation. But you are not alone, and there are both ways to get better and people who can help. Reading this book may be the first step on the journey to recovery, and with some help and support, life can improve.

3

The bio, the psycho and the social: explanatory models of CFS/ME

On the basis of what we have said already, we can see that scientists and doctors have yet to find a single cause of CFS/ME. This doesn't mean that in time and with more research one won't be found, but for the moment it appears CFS/ME is much more complex than just a viral infection. Many researchers have put forward models, or theories, about the development of the disorder, and in this chapter we will focus on one model in an effort to present the body of research in CFS/ME in a coherent way. However, this information can also be used in support of other models that we will explore in the next chapter.

The biopsychosocial model

The biopsychosocial model was developed by the psychiatrist George Engel in the late 1970s and early 1980s. In 1977 he published a paper in the prestigious journal *Science* in which he stated: 'The dominant model of disease today is biomedical, and it leaves no room within this framework for the social, psychological, and behavioural dimensions of illness.' In other words, he was somewhat frustrated with the rather simplistic view of the patient as flesh and blood; we all interact with other people and our environment in our own, individual way, and these aspects of our world can be important, if not vital, to our health and well-being. In a further article, Dr Engel presented a case study of a 55-year-old married salesman whom he presented pseudonymously as 'Mr Glover'. Mr Glover has a history of heart disease – he had a heart attack six months previously – and has started to feel a growing pressure within his chest and aching in his left arm. However, he dismisses his bodily sensations as wind, muscle strain and emotional tension, 'not another heart attack', even though the sensations did remind him of his previous myocardial infarction (heart attack). Instead Mr Glover, being the conscientious fellow he is and perhaps worried about how another attack will affect his job, busies himself quite frantically with getting his work in order between bouts of sitting quietly to let the sensations pass. It is not until his employer notices his behaviour that he is persuaded to go to hospital. Once at the hospital the medics follow prescribed procedures, and even though this causes pain and discomfort, Mr Glover doesn't feel able to protest, even though he can see the doctors struggling. Eventually they request further assistance from more experienced colleagues. These circumstances lead Mr Glover to lose consciousness, but fortunately the medical team is able to resuscitate him. In the article Dr Engel unpicks the influences and interactions that resulted in Mr Glover's case. If we break this down into the biopsychosocial model's components we can see the following factors at play:

bio – the underlying biological processes that led to Mr Glover's heart disease and subsequent attacks;

psycho – the personal, psychological and behavioural characteristics of Mr Glover. At first he ignored the chest pain and other symptoms and attributed them to innocuous causes. Then he was more concerned with getting his affairs in order and so delayed going to hospital, which exacerbated his symptoms;

social – the wider influences on a situation from others, such as family, friends, doctors, policy-makers, government, and more general social, political and cultural influences. Mr Glover's boss finally convinced him to take his symptoms seriously and escorted him to the hospital; without her, he might have delayed too long and the damage could have been permanent. Also, the cultural norms at the time – remember this was a case from the late 1970s published in 1980 – shaped Mr Glover's inability to criticize the medics even when he could clearly see they were labouring over his treatment. If he had been more comfortable in stating his pain and distress, the doctors might have sought more experienced colleagues more quickly.

Dr Engel specifically chose a medical, rather than a psychiatric case, to exemplify his theory. He wanted to show the academic and medical community that even an acute illness such as a myocardial infarction can be affected by psychological and social aspects of a person's life, not just illnesses that clearly have a psychiatric origin.

When thinking about CFS/ME it has been proposed that the biopsychosocial model may be a useful way to explain the condition. It is relevant here to note that those who champion this model more usually come from a psychiatric or psychological background, which is not surprising, as Dr Engel states: 'How physicians approach patients and the problems they present is very much influenced by the conceptual models in relationship to which their knowledge and experience are organized.' Thus an immunologist may see someone with CFS/ME and focus on her immune system's function, whereas a psychologist may see the same person and believe she needs to find better coping strategies to deal with the condition.

The 'bio'

Let's look at how the biopsychosocial model can be applied to CFS/ME. As we saw in Chapter 1, numerous viruses have been associated with CFS/ME over time, not just Epstein-Barr virus (EBV) but also Q fever and Ross River virus and the human herpesviruses 6 (HHV-6) and 7 (HHV-7). Interestingly, in 2006 a research group in California found that of their group of people with CFS/ME who also had positive test results for HHV-6 and EBV, 9 out of 12 responded well to treatment with the anti-viral drug valganciclovir. Indeed improvement in symptoms following the treatment led to a return to work and/or full-time activities. However, as we discussed in previous chapters, because there still is no consistent evidence that a virus is the culprit, proponents of the biopsychosocial model for CFS/ME state that a virus or other type of infection may be a 'triggering' event but not the complete cause of the illness. (In this model, triggering events would not necessarily have to be a virus but could be a bacterial infection, exposure to dangerous chemicals such as pesticides, physical trauma such as surgery or a car accident and even a traumatic life event such as the death of a spouse, partner or loved one.)

The 'psycho'

In terms of the 'psycho' – the psychological and individual person factors – in this model for CFS/ME, there have been many personality traits suggested by numerous researchers over the years. This is a hotly debated topic, and if you take the argument to the nth degree, it may appear that people with CFS/ME are responsible for their condition. Was Mr Glover above to blame for his heart attack? No, of course not. Could he have dealt with his symptoms differently? Perhaps, but you cannot take the person out of his context, so he dealt with the situation as best he could under the circumstances at the time. Therefore in Dr Engel's original model the psychological dimension was not included to put the onus on the patient, rather to understand more fully the complex nature of human health and illness. With regard to CFS/ME, early studies stated that people with the condition had higher levels of the personality trait 'neuroticism'. However, this doesn't mean someone is neurotic per se, rather personality theory implies that people who report high levels of neuroticism are more susceptible to anxiety, low mood, lack of contentment and sometimes anger – but do bear in mind that personalities are not defined by one trait. Also, the trait of neuroticism includes a tendency towards perfectionism (always wanting to get things 'right'), the fear of making mistakes and having very high personal standards. However, these early findings were not always confirmed by later studies. For instance, in comparison to a fatiguing disorder where the cause is clear (rheumatoid arthritis), there were no major differences in questionnaire results for perfectionism, which is a personality trait seen to be related to neuroticism in the scientific literature. This means that the higher levels of neuroticism and related traits found in people with illnesses such as CFS/ME may have been due to the condition – so rather than assuming that people with these traits are more likely to become ill with CFS/ME, it may be that fatiguing conditions cause people to be more perfectionistic. Without studies that measure these traits over time, especially before and after people become ill, it is impossible to conclude that neuroticism and perfectionism lead directly to the development of CFS/ME.

People with CFS/ME have been observed to have other personality characteristics. For example, in comparison to individuals with psychiatric disorders and chronic conditions with a known cause, those with CFS/ME have been shown to be driven towards direct action and achievement, a trait the researchers called 'action proneness'. Perhaps tellingly, however, in this study people with CFS/ME had similar levels of action proneness to those with chronic pain conditions, which suggests the possibility that these two long-term, invisible conditions may develop in the same way. These findings have been supported by further research that assessed not self-reported action proneness, rather ratings on this trait by the significant other – such as wife, husband, partner or even carer – of those with CFS/ME. This corroboration is important as it can be difficult for us all, whether we have a fatiguing condition or not, to recall the past accurately. This research showed that in comparison to healthy people there were similar levels of action proneness for people with CFS/ME as for individuals with another condition – fibromyalgia – where the exact cause is uncertain. This again implies that perhaps a personality driven by action may predispose people to develop chronic illness.

Furthermore, on the topic of heightened 'action', when asked 'What were you like before you became ill?', individuals with CFS/ME were found to regard themselves as being more 'hard-driving' than people in good health. Yet again in this research the ratings from people with CFS/ME were similar to those from people with IBS, which is again another condition with an uncertain underlying cause. A group of psychiatrists and researchers at the Institute of Psychiatry in London also looked at activity, but in this case physical activity. The researchers in this group have a special interest in the epidemiology (distribution of a disease, who it affects and where) and aetiology (cause of a disease) of CFS/ME. They therefore carefully designed a study that looked at a large group of nearly 3,000 people from birth to 53 years old, to find out if those who developed CFS/ME differed in any way from people who did not. Interestingly people with CFS/ME did not experience any more childhood illnesses or allergies than those who remained healthy throughout life. But in childhood and early adulthood, people who were later diagnosed with CFS/ME were on average more physically active and of lower body weight. Tellingly (and this may be the key to the 'psycho' in the biopsychosocial model), once these individuals started to have symptoms of fatigue they did not rest and give themselves a break but instead carried on with their exercise routines.

So it seems that even when people experience symptoms, those who end up with CFS/ME push through and try to ignore their discomfort. Like Mr Glover in Dr Engel's example, this may be because of concern for others such as our partners and families, not wanting to let people down, feeling responsible for getting things done and so on. This may also be why in early studies of personality and CFS/ME, people appeared to have higher levels of neuroticism and perfectionism: the concept of neuroticism includes worry, hence worrying about letting people down may have been on people's minds; and perfectionism can be related to high personal standards, such as doing the very best you can even in the face of ill health. Taken together, this body of knowledge implies that those who become ill with long-term fatiguing conditions – not just CFS/ME but also related conditions such as fibromyalgia and IBS – were motivated, determined and ambitious people who did not give their bodies space to recover in times of ill health. In terms of the biopsychosocial model this is important when taken together with the 'bio' (the viral or other type of strain on the immune system). The picture that is emerging is one in which, when some people get ill with an acute illness such as a virus or even experience a traumatic event, they carry on regardless, even in the face of deteriorating health. Indeed in a study in which interviewees were asked about how their illness began, those with CFS/ME cited infection, 'doing too much', stressful circumstances, physical vulnerability, personality and neglecting health. Interestingly they also reported an initial period of recovery after an acute episode of illness, known as 'phased' onset. This interval in which health had improved was followed by a descent into chronic illness, which the interviewees attributed to overactivity, immediate return to work after the original period of illness, and occupational stress and daily hassles before symptoms started.

Next we will look at these more 'social' aspects of stress, daily hassles and wider social and cultural factors, and relate these to Dr Engel's biopsychosocial model in CFS/ME.

The 'social'

Dr Engel felt it was very important, in his model, to think about the wider aspects of life that may affect health. We have seen both in the case of Mr Glover and in the academic literature that there are certain personality characteristics and ways of behaving that may influence health and illness. But there are also things about our daily lives, perhaps the jobs we have and our relationships with others, that may edge us towards illness. If we think of health as a continuum, it is unlikely that, especially as we get older, we are 100 per cent healthy or 100 per cent ill (which would mean death). So we vary over our lives in terms of how healthy/ill we are. If we think about health and illness as a continuum, these two states of being are polar opposites – most people lie somewhere between them.

In this sense we could conceptualize health and illness as a number of things, including functioning, well-being, symptoms or lack of symptoms and so on, which has been done in many studies. When thinking about the biopsychosocial model it is not to say that if you are highly 'action prone' you will become unwell or your functioning in the world will decrease, rather that when this trait is combined with a nasty viral infection such as glandular fever, and you go back to a highly stressful job and at the same time your mother becomes ill and you need to fight social services to place her in residential care, then the collective weight of all these pressures may just push the continuum from health towards illness.

When considering the 'social' in the biopsychosocial model, life events may be an important area to consider. In the late 1960s the psychiatrists Thomas Holmes and Richard Rahe observed that major incidents seemed to affect people's health. In order to 'operational-ize' or standardize their impact on someone's health they devised a list of 43 events suggested by the doctors' clinical experience. Nearly 400 people then rated the amount these events affected their lives. An updated list was then compiled so that the most severe events had higher scores attached (for example, 'death of spouse' has a value of 100 whereas 'Christmas' has a value of 12), with the idea that although a minor event such as Christmas may not affect health, perhaps the death of a partner, trouble at work and then Christmas on top of it all would lead someone to become ill. This scale has now been used in countless research studies and it is a generally accepted principle that life events can – but of course may not always – move someone's health continuum towards illness.

In terms of CFS/ME, researchers from the Academic Unit of Psychiatry and Behavioural Sciences at the School of Medicine of the University of Leeds looked at 64 patients with CFS/ME who had been referred to the Infectious Diseases/Liaison Psychiatry Fatigue clinic, and 64 people who were the same sex and age as the people with CFS/ME and lived locally. The researchers found that at two time-points – 12 months and 3 months before symptoms started – the people with CFS/ME had experienced more 'life events' than the healthy people who acted as a comparison group. A similar trend was found in another study that looked at a year leading up to the onset of illness: those with CFS/ME had more marital separations and conflicts at work than healthy people of the same age and sex. This study also observed that the greater the frequency of negative life events increased, the closer people came to becoming ill. Interestingly the number of infections the participants in this study cited also increased in the preceding four months before their health became poor. But it's not all doom and gloom! Life events can also be positive and have been shown to assist recovery in those with CFS/ME – for example, the birth of a new family member. In fact positive life events needn't be major occurrences – small things such as gifts, invitations, unexpected meetings with friends or even a beautiful day can act as positive events and be beneficial.

In addition to the individual negative events that have been shown to be influential in CFS/ME, continual trauma has also been linked to the development of the condition. In a study with nearly 800 people with CFS/ME, sexual abuse in childhood was associated with fatigue in adulthood, as was the total number of abusive events. In comparison with fatiguing disorders where there is a known cause such as rheumatoid arthritis and multiple sclerosis, researchers found that individuals with medically unexplained conditions such as CFS/ME and fibro-myalgia had higher rates of emotional abuse, emotional neglect and physical abuse. A proportion of the individuals with CFS/ME and fibromyalgia experienced this abuse throughout their lives – that is, the abuse did not occur as isolated incidents and was most often com-mitted by close family members or partners. These findings have been seen as quite controversial, but it is relevant to take into account the experiences of people who have reported abuse – this is not to say that everyone with CFS/ME has had these experiences or that everyone who has faced abuse will develop a fatiguing condition; abuse simply might be yet another aspect of someone's life that will nudge her or him along the continuum from health to illness.

The final area that we will explore with regard to the 'social' aspect of the biopsychosocial model is daily hassles. In terms of scientific research, as opposed to our lay understanding of hassles, daily hassles can be categorized into seven different groups (with examples): inner concerns (regrets over past decisions and feeling lonely), financial concerns (worries about not having enough money for basic neces-sities and concerns about getting into debt), time pressures (worries about having too many things to do and not getting enough sleep), work hassles (job dissatisfaction and not liking colleagues), environ-mental hassles (pollution and crime), family hassles (being overloaded with housework and problems with children) and finally health has-sles (concerns about medical treatment and physical illness). Just read-ing this list is probably making you feel hassled. Also, if these things weren't on your mind before you had CFS/ME, they most probably would be once symptoms start, so if the examples seem familiar then you are certainly not alone. Indeed researchers from the Netherlands found this to be the case when they compared 177 people with either CFS/ME or fibromyalgia to 26 people with rheumatoid arthritis and 26 people with multiple sclerosis. The team asked all these groups to record the number of daily hassles they experienced and also the level of distress this caused two to four months after they had been diag-nosed with their respective conditions. What was interesting in this study was that those with CFS/ME and fibromyalgia reported higher numbers of daily hassles when compared to people with the other illnesses, even though rheumatoid arthritis and multiple sclerosis are also fatiguing and debilitating conditions. In fact whereas the rheumatoid arthritis and multiple sclerosis groups reported a range of daily hassles across the categories, the types of hassles people with CFS/ME and fibromyalgia stated clustered more on the 'covert' or private hassles (such as dissatisfaction with oneself, insecurity and a lack of social recognition) rather than the 'overt' or public hassles (such as work and environmental worries). It seems plausible that the reason for this difference was more 'social' than 'psycho', and related to stigma and delegitimation (that is, people such as doctors, friends and family dismissing your condition), although the authors of this study did not discuss this explicitly.

There is a large body of scientific evidence showing that people with CFS/ME are stigmatized. Stigma is a culturally engendered phenomenon that makes people feel different – in a negative way – from the rest of society on the basis of perceived characteristics. People can be stigmatized on the basis of overtly observable features such as skin colour and gender, or more internal aspects such as beliefs and ideologies (for example, their religion). The important point about stigma is that it is the *perceptions* from others that create damaging experiences, and of course perceptions and attitudes can be very ingrained indeed.

In the 1990s the medical anthropologist Norma Ware – now based in the Department of Global Health and Social Medicine at the prestigious Harvard Medical School – published a number of studies looking at the experience and illness-course of those with CFS/ME in relation to the cultural and social elements that affected these experiences. Stigma was a common theme that Ware found in the interviews she carried out with people who had CFS/ME, who often had their symptoms trivialized by others. This trivialization was not only by family, friends, colleagues and so on – people with no formal medical qualifications – but also medical professionals such as doctors, nurses and health workers. The absence of proper legitimation of their symptoms led the people in Ware's studies to experience further distress over and above the pain and fatigue caused by the disorder. She illustrated this with some very powerful quotes, including from one individual who stated that she would have preferred to have been diagnosed with cancer and its associated progression, prognosis and treatment options – even if the cancer were to be terminal – rather than the uncertainty, delegitimation and resulting 'torment' CFS/ME had produced.

Hence it is not surprising that the people in studies of daily hassles often report greater levels of private worry such as dissatisfaction with oneself, insecurity and a lack of social recognition, because the social and cultural environment may lead them to feel unworthy, vulnerable and that they have little support from others. Therefore the 'social' aspect of Dr Engel's biopsychosocial model does appear relevant when considering the progression of CFS/ME.

Summary and conclusion

Before we move on to the next chapter and start to discuss additional models relevant to CFS/ME, it is important to appreciate that
the research cited above was not specifically carried out to 'prove'
the biopsychosocial model – it can just as easily be used to support
other models that attempt to explain the development of CFS/ME.
This book does not seek to defend any one model; rather its aim is to
present the information so that you can get a clearer understanding of
CFS/ME and use this to improve your or your loved one's life. Many
people reject the biopsychosocial model because it has been linked to
psychological therapies (which we will discuss in Chapter 6), but this
was not Dr Engel's intent when he devised his theory. We imagine
he would have been just as aghast at the simplification of CFS/ME
into a purely psychological illness as he was at the very reductionist
biomedical model at the time. The introduction of a model that takes
into account not only the biological and physiological components of
a disease but also the psychological and wider social aspects of health
and illness has been an important step forward for many illnesses. The
issue with CFS/ME may be that we are still unsure as to the precise
physical mechanisms, which could be why this conceptualization of
the illness has been rejected by some.

4

Not all in the mind: current physiological research

As we saw in the previous chapter, Dr Engel was frustrated with the prevailing view and teaching of medicine during his time as a doctor in the sense that it only focused on the physical body and ignored the other influences on a human being such as their behaviours, interactions with others and also the impact of the wider social world. However, this was not always the case in medicine, and indeed current models of health and illness have started to take into account how the mind and body interact. In this chapter we will explore some of the models that show us *how* the mind and body are 'networked' and therefore cannot be viewed as separate entities.

The mind, the body and stress

Although Dr Engel felt that medicine had become too 'reductionist' – reducing a person and his or her health to basic biological and chemical elements – this had not always been the case. Ancient civilizations in Greece and Egypt recognized the impact of nutrition, personal and family situation and even 'stress' on a person's health. When medicine began to evolve very quickly with the introduction of technology in the nineteenth century, the discipline tried to imitate science by looking at disease in terms of cause and effect. While these advances were incredibly important and increased life expectancy greatly, there was the drawback that now the 'art' of medical practice was sidelined – doctors treated the *disease* rather than the *person*.

However, in the later stages of the twentieth century and certainly within this century there has been a great deal of theorizing and subsequent research that has shown the interaction between the mind and body, or person, and his or her health. The Austrian endocrinologist Hans Seyle was a very important figure in this field – it was he who coined the term 'stress' and made the link between psychological or emotional reactions, physiological processes and disease. However, a 'stressor' – something that causes stress – does not have to be psychological in the way that is viewed currently, but can be physical, such as a demanding environment or toxin. In fact it has only been in the past 50 years or so that 'stress' has been in everyday language; before this it was more an expression used in physics to imply strain brought about by force – although we can see how this does transpose to our understanding of stress now.

In 1950 Dr Seyle published his observations in the seminal paper, 'Stress and the General Adaptation Syndrome', in the *British Medical Journal*. His theory was based on a considerable body of work – a bit of a workaholic, he was often seen working up to 14 hours a day and during holidays and weekends – and central to it was the concept of 'homeostasis'. Homeostasis is the need for a system or organism to maintain equilibrium – that is, balance. A simple example of this is temperature control (the mechanisms are complex but let's put that to one side for the moment): if our bodies overheat we sweat to keep cool, and when we are too cold we shiver to generate heat. Dr Seyle devised his General Adaptation Syndrome (GAS) as three stages, extending from the 'fight or flight' response to danger. When we are presented with a threat – for our ancestors this may have been a lion on the plains of Africa but for us may be dealing with our boss on a Monday morning – our bodies react in such a way as to give us the best chance of survival. To be able to come out alive in an encounter with a lion – or our boss – our nervous and endocrine systems will release a multitude of signals and hormones to induce numerous physiological changes. For instance, our blood flow will surge to charge our muscles to allow us to run as fast as we can; our pupils will dilate so that we can see as clearly as possible; and the sugars and fats in our blood will increase to provide us with as much energy as possible. In GAS, Seyle termed this the 'alarm response' stage. In the second stage, 'resistance', these physiological changes are reversed and our bodies return to homeostasis – that is, they adapt. However, if the body cannot adapt because of genetic factors or the continued presence of a stressor, we reach the third stage, 'exhaustion', and it is this stage that can lead to ill health. Although the association between stress and disease may seem obvious to us now, Seyle's work was groundbreaking and he was nominated for a Nobel Prize on many occasions, though sadly he never received it.

Subsequent work has shown exactly what physiological alterations happen when we are confronted with a stressful situation (that is, in the 'alarm response' stage of the GAS model), both in our endocrine systems and our autonomic nervous system (ANS). Before we move on to the research studies, let's start with a quick recap. The endocrine system is made up of numerous glands that secrete hormones. These hormones enable the body to maintain homeostasis and also regulate metabolism, growth, sleep and even mood. The ANS is basically a type of control system that influences heart and respiratory rates, digestion, pupil dilation, sweating and the need to urinate, among other functions. The hypothalamus – an area of the brain located just above the brain stem – is an important part of both the endocrine and autonomic nervous systems. Some of the hormones the hypothalamus releases kick-start – or deter – the pituitary gland secreting hormones. This process in turn influences the adrenal glands, and the sequential relationship between these structures is known as the 'hypothalamic–pituitary–adrenal axis', or 'HPA axis' for short. The HPA axis is essentially 'activated' in times of acute stress (such as the lion/boss situation), when it acts as a feedback loop, releasing or inhibiting the production of hormones to regulate the functions important in fight or flight.

This process is an excellent way for us to stay safe from the lion (by staying very still and hiding or running as fast as we can) or dealing with our boss (by thinking on our feet or hiding behind the water cooler), but problems can occur if our bodies cannot revert back to a state of homeostasis and physiological balance. In Dr Seyle's GAS model this would be the third phase, 'exhaustion'. There is now quite a body of evidence showing that at least some people with CFS/ME have an altered HPA axis, which implies that they couldn't reach homeostasis in the 'resistance' stage of the GAS model and so are in a state of exhaustion. A number of these studies have looked at levels of cortisol, a steroid hormone that plays a role in various bodily systems, such as the circulatory, nervous and immune system, metabolism and importantly the stress response. Testing levels of cortisol can demonstrate the function of the pituitary and adrenal glands. However, the amount of cortisol released varies throughout the day: in the morning it rises sharply, then gradually diminishes during the day to rise again in later afternoon. In the late evening cortisol levels will decrease once again and should be at their lowest in the middle of the night. This fluctuation is linked to our sleep/wake cycle – known as the circadian rhythm – and hence if this pattern has gone off course, it can be an indication of a dysfunction of the HPA axis. Overall levels of cortisol can also indicate disease – abnormally high levels denote Cushing's disease and lower than normal levels can suggest Addison's disease.

In a study published in 2004, 56 people who had been referred to the specialist CFS/ME clinic at King's College Hospital in London had their cortisol levels tested just after waking up in the morning.

This 'cortisol awakening response' is seen to be a good measure of HPA axis function – cortisol levels rise around 50–60 per cent after waking and remain high for about an hour. It is also relatively easy to test for because cortisol can be traced in saliva – participants could take their samples at home and simply post the sample tubes to the research centre. In comparison to 35 healthy people, those with CFS/ME had lower levels of cortisol ten minutes after waking up and also after being awake for an hour. However, not all studies looking at the HPA axis have shown these sorts of problems, which may be because there are different 'sub-groups' that have all been diagnosed with CFS/ME (a topic we will discuss in Chapter 10). Nevertheless there is clear evidence of HPA axis irregularities in people who have CFS/ME, which suggests that their systems have not been able to revert back to a state of balance, or homeostasis. In the GAS model then, those with CFS/ME are stuck in the stage of exhaustion.

Psychoneuroimmunology (PNI)

While Dr Seyle's careful observations and experimental studies were undoubtedly important in the evolution of our understanding of the links between the mind and the body and the influence of stress, some of his assertions were incorrect and he didn't unveil all the processes involved in the stress response. One key area missed was immunology, which is perhaps unsurprising considering that Seyle was an endocrinologist not an immunologist. An area of study that does look at the immune system in relation to stress is 'psychoneuroimmunology' (PNI). PNI can be broken down into its constituent parts:

psycho – here 'psycho' refers most to the behaviour of people, but this is of course affected by our thoughts, beliefs and personalities;
neuro – not just the nervous system but also endocrine system, which acts in a similar way to the nervous system as it sends signals throughout the body, though the effects from endocrine signals last much longer – hours or even weeks – compared to the immediate responses of the nervous system;
immunology – the main purpose of the immune system is to protect us from pathogens, such as viruses and bacteria, that may cause disease. The really impressive thing about the immune system is that it is adaptive – it can tailor its first non-specific response to a pathogen so that next time the virus or bacterium invades, a faster and stronger attack can be mounted.

Hence those in the field of PNI investigate the relationships and interactions between our behaviour and the nervous, endocrine and immune systems. The term 'psychoneuroimmunology' was coined in 1980 by Robert Ader, an American psychologist and academic who spent his career at the University of Rochester (Dr Ader died in 2011). Tellingly, this was the same institution Dr Engel was based at for a significant proportion of his career. It is often fascinating to look beyond the publications of scientists and academics and dig a little deeper into their history and context to see exactly how ideas emerged. Hence Engel was heavily influential in the development of Ader's research, and in 1998 Ader stated that the reason he'd stayed at Rochester for his entire career was in part due to Engel's encouragement. But PNI was a somewhat accidental discovery for Ader when he observed that it was possible to 'trick' the immune system while he was working on a series of animal studies. He then worked closely with the microbiologist Nicholas Cohen, and in 1975 the two researchers stated, based on their studies of immunosuppression, that there was undoubtedly a link between the brain and the immune system.

The field of PNI has now elicited thousands of studies that show the relationship between the brain and immune system. Ader and Cohen's work was mainly looking at how psychological and behavioural processes suppress, or dampen down, the immune system and so leave us more vulnerable to infection. Many researchers have followed up and extended this work, in particular the husband and wife duo Professors Ronald Glaser and Janice Kiecolt-Glaser. Both are based within the Institute for Behavioral Medicine Research at the Ohio State University College of Medicine, where Ronald Glaser is Director. They have produced a body of PNI work since the early 1990s and each published hundreds of scientific journal articles. They make a pretty auspicious pairing for PNI research when it comes to their educational background: Janice Kiecolt-Glaser's expertise is within psychology and psychiatry whereas Ronald Glaser has medical qualifications in molecular virology, immunology and genetics. It would be harder to find a more fitting duo to conduct PNI research.

Throughout their work, Professors Glaser and Kiecolt-Glaser have been particularly interested in the impact of stress on the immunological function of caregivers, specifically adults who look after a relative with dementia or Alzheimer's disease. In a study that recruited participants from the local Alzheimer's Disease Association support groups, 32 people who cared for their spouse with either Alzheimer's disease, dementia, Parkinson's disease or Huntington's disease volunteered for the study. To compare the immune response to an influenza vaccination, 32 people who were the same sex, age and had similar levels of income but who were not carers were also recruited into the study. Notably the carers spent, on average, more than eight hours a day caring for their spouse or partner, so the daily care requirement was quite high. Blood samples were collected a week before the flu vaccine, and then at four weeks post-inoculation and a further three and six months after the injection. This was so that the researchers could look for the immune response that would be expected from a vaccination. The results showed that only 12 of the caregivers had an appropriate immune response compared to 21 of the non-carers four weeks after the vaccine, even though the groups had similar levels of immunity to the flu before the testing. This was a statistically significant – that is, meaningful – finding and showed PNI in a real-world setting, not simply in the animal models of early PNI work.

But it is not just the inability to fight infection that 'stress' appears to influence – it seems that the body's capacity to heal wounds is also affected by psychological stress and responsibilities. A further study by the husband and wife team looked again at people who were caring for a relative with Alzheimer's disease, but this time only female caregivers. Thirteen female carers were matched in terms of age and income with non-carers, and had a small wound of 3.5 mm made with a 'punch biopsy' (basically a large needle), placed just under the elbow. A week after the biopsy the researchers took photos of the wound every 2–8 days to track healing, and only stopped assessing the women's arms when the wound had completely healed. On average the wounds on the women who were looking after their relatives with dementia took 49 days to heal, whereas those on the women who didn't have this role healed after only 39 days. This ten-day difference was statistically meaningful. Additionally the researchers drew blood samples from the women to look at immunological function. They found that the carers produced fewer cytokines than the non-carers. As cytokines are molecules released by the immune system that help the healing process by stimulating collagen and connective tissue, among numerous other activities, this demonstrated a possible mechanism for why those with caring responsibilities had longer healing times. If we think back to Chapter 3 and the discussion of 'daily hassles', caring for a relative with a demanding illness such as Alzheimer's disease could cause you to have many worries, including those of 'time pressure' and 'family hassles'. Indeed it has been shown that people who provide long-term care for loved ones with dementia report high levels of stress.

Therefore we are starting to understand *how* the mind and body are interrelated and why the 'psycho' and the 'social' of Dr Engel's model are influential in health and illness.

Finally on the topic of PNI, this model can also act as a loop. To give an example of this, let's think about a hypothetical person called Maggie. Maggie has a part-time job and three young children, and has been married for 13 years. Over a period of 12 months her father's health deteriorates and she has to battle with social services to provide him with home help and eventually residential care. Maggie's husband helps as much as he can, but he has a very demanding job and works full-time. Then one of the kids picks up glandular fever from someone at school and Maggie also contracts the virus. Maggie's employer is understanding at first, but after she has to take an extended period of time off he gets rather anxious and puts pressure on her to return because his small business cannot cope with a key employee off sick for more than a few days. Maggie's boss cites the recession as the reason – he doesn't want Maggie to feel bad but she does feel guilty about letting him down. Because Maggie is so exhausted from the illness she also feels guilty about 'not being a good mother' and so tries to ignore her symptoms and carry on with all the kids' activities. However, she finds it difficult to sleep because she's constantly worried about her dad and what to do about her job – if she gives it up the family will struggle financially. She goes back to work and tries to nap before the kids get back from school, and in doing this she doesn't find the time to make herself lunch or do the exercise classes she used to fit in. Eventually Maggie's body can take no more and she has to go back to her doctor and ask for help. From this example we can see how a carefully balanced life can quickly go out of kilter with major life-stress (father's illness), daily hassles (looking after the children, worries over work and money) and acute infection followed by the demise of behaviours that maintain health, such as sleep, diet and exercise, which are known to help the immune system. The end result may be chronic immune activation and a cycle of ill health.

Bio(psychosocial) model

Michael Maes, a neuropsychiatrist based in Bangkok, has published several scientific papers that focus much more on the biological and physiological aspects of CFS/ME. In his 2010 paper, 'Chronic Fatigue Syndrome: Harvey and Wessely's (Bio)psychosocial Model Versus a Bio(psychosocial) Model Based on Inflammatory and Oxidative and

Nitrosative Stress Pathways', he reconceptualized the biopsycho-social model that we outlined in Chapter 3. Dr Maes insisted in this article that most of the biological factors that have been associated with CFS/ME over the years were ignored by proponents of the bio-psychosocial model, or simply characterized as triggering factors rather than key aspects of the illness. Instead it has been on the behavioural responses to symptoms, such as bedrest and limiting activity, that researchers and doctors who use biopsychosocial model as a basis for understanding CFS/ME have concentrated their attention. Therefore Maes referred to this as the '(bio)psychosocial' model, because the most important areas were seen to be the 'psycho' and the 'social'. Furthermore, he presented this model in a new way, with the 'bio' at the centre of the theory – that is, the bio(psychosocial) model of CFS/ME. You may be wondering, 'Well all right, but why does this matter?' The answer is two-fold. First, CFS/ME is still a highly stigma-tized illness (see Chapter 3), with echoes of past assertions that those with CFS/ME were/are 'malingerers', only have 'yuppie flu' and 'It's all in the mind' – so not having 'a real illness'. This new version of the biopsychosocial model firmly puts at its forefront the biological and physiological abnormalities that have been discovered in CFS/ME, and therefore confirms CFS/ME as a very real and debilitating condition. Second, the (bio)psychosocial model has, unsurprisingly, resulted in predominately psychological and behavioural treatments (we will outline these in Chapter 6). While these have been shown to be effec-tive in some people with CFS/ME, they are not acceptable to everyone with the condition because many do not see the justification for psy-chological approaches for the treatment of a physical condition. But if we take on board the bio(psychosocial) model of CFS/ME, this leads us to concentrate much more on the physiological processes underlying the illness, some of which may respond to targeted treatment.

One example of a physiological mechanism that could be treated on an individual basis is mitochondrial dysfunction. The mitochondria are known as the 'power houses' of cells as they provide every living cell in the body with energy. This is achieved via an intricate chemical process. However, the mitochondria can stop working properly due to genetic mutations, infections or other environmental factors such as drugs and toxins. Recently there has been interest in the role of mito-chondrial function in CFS/ME because one sign that something is not working properly in the mitochondria can be reduced energy. Sarah Myhill, a private GP based in rural Wales, has been an advocate of the importance of mitochondria in CFS/ME for many years, and has been treating people on this basis. Her clinic has published three studies based on an audit of 138 of her patients. It is useful to bear in mind that a clinical audit is different from a research study with preset aims – audits are a more exploratory way to look at data, and because they are carried out with information from a clinical setting, they will not have the rigorous controls in place that research studies should have. Nevertheless audits give us important findings, and often these will be double-checked through research studies.

Dr Myhill's work illustrated that those with CFS/ME did indeed have observable mitochondrial dysfunction. Interestingly, in the published work she showed that mitochondrial dysfunction appeared to be associated with the severity of symptoms – people with greater mitochondrial dysfunction were more ill. This is potentially a quite important finding because it implies a clear relationship between how well the mitochondria are working and the level of illness someone might have. There needs to be a great deal more work in this area to find out exactly what's going wrong in the mitochondria in people with CFS/ME, and to this end the Medical Research Council in the UK has funded a study based in the Institute of Ageing and Chronic Disease at the University of Liverpool. This study is specifically looking at mitochondrial function in the muscles of people with CFS/ME. Work of this type shows the increased attention physiology is now attracting in this condition, which perhaps supports Dr Maes' new conceptualization of the bio(psychosocial) model of CFS/ME.

Summary and conclusion

In this chapter we have looked at the interaction between the mind and the body and the impact that stress can have on us all. We also explored some quite complex physiological models that have been developed to explain what may be going on in the bodies of people with CFS/ME. The jury is still out regarding which one is correct, but from the discussion of a few – though certainly not all – models presented to explain the condition, the hope is that you can see how much physiological research is being conducted. In the next chapter we will move away from this technical information and focus on the more practical issue of what to do when you first become ill.

5

What to do when you first get ill: symptoms and diagnosis

CFS/ME is a highly variable condition, meaning that everyone's experience of it differs. This can, first, make it difficult for people to describe their illness – it often feels as though there are so many things going on at once. But, second, this variability can also make it tricky for doctors to diagnose CFS/ME. In this chapter we will look in more detail at some of the key symptoms in CFS/ME and the research behind them, before moving on to look more closely at how the condition is diagnosed.

Symptoms

Fatigue

By far the most common symptom in CFS/ME is fatigue (unsurprisingly) but, like pain, fatigue can occur in many different forms. If we think about pain for a minute, when you go to the doctor's and say you're in pain she will usually ask if it is a stabbing, throbbing or even pressured pain. Although your doctor may not have asked you a similar question about fatigue, there is evidence that fatigue is not simply 'tiredness'. Researchers have looked at fatigue in detail and found that people with CFS/ME report five different types of fatigue:

1 post-exertional fatigue;
2 energy fatigue;
3 wired fatigue;
4 brain fog;
5 flu-like fatigue.

Post-exertional fatigue or malaise

Post-exertional fatigue – sometimes called post-exertional malaise – is tiredness that occurs after mental and physical activity. This is a key symptom in CFS/ME, so much so that in the case definitions of CFS/

ME, post-exertional malaise is a separate symptom. The important difference between post-exertional fatigue and the tiredness that healthy people would feel after activity is that the severity of the fatigue in those with CFS/ME is far greater than would be expected from the nature of the activity. For instance, simply walking to a corner shop would not usually be difficult for healthy people and would not make them feel worn out, but for people with CFS/ME that small amount of exertion may affect them so much that they would need to lie down for the rest of the day. Gerald says he feels all right when he's not doing too much but tires very easily:

> The big thing, the thing that really spoils your life, is what I call a lack of stamina. I don't like this concept of chronic fatigue. I'm not tired all the time, sometimes I'm not tired at all. If I do nothing I often feel pretty well; as soon as I start doing something it tires me too quickly. (Gerald)

A research group at the Workwell Foundation (a charity based in Ripon, California, USA) has been investigating post-exertional fatigue for a number of years. In 2013 the group, led by Drs Christopher Snell and Mark VanNess, published an important study that clearly demonstrated the existence of post-exertional fatigue. In this study the researchers compared 51 women with CFS/ME to ten healthy women on an exercise task. This task was carried out on a stationary exercise bike and the women were asked to pedal for as long as they could manage. During the pedalling, breath samples and heart-rate measurements were taken so that the researchers could be sure the women were at 'peak effort', meaning exercising as hard as they could. Importantly, the healthy women in this study were not super-fit individuals but sedentary people who did not exercise regularly or do more than 30 minutes of moderate physical activity most days of the week. During this first exercise task the women with CFS/ME and the healthy, albeit sedentary women performed pretty much the same. But – and this is the telling aspect of the study – when the women were asked to come back 24 hours later and do the task again, differences were found. One day after the first pedalling attempt, the women with CFS/ME found it much harder to reach their previous levels of peak effort than they had the day before. For the healthy women, 24 hours was plenty of time to recover and do the pedalling again with the same intensity. The researchers calculated that by using this two-day 'cardiopulmonary exercise testing', people with CFS/ME could be differentiated from healthy people with an accuracy of 95 per cent. This study, and some previous work that this research team carried out, shows objective evidence for post-exertional fatigue. This type of exercise testing may also be used as a diagnostic procedure at some point in the future.

Energy fatigue

Energy fatigue is when you simply feel too tired to do even the most simple of tasks – taking a shower, putting some washing on or making food. This type of fatigue can make it very hard for people to care for themselves and others, to work, go to school and even have relationships. Sarah explains how it can be difficult to do all the everyday things we need to do when having CFS/ME:

> I feel all right at the moment. I'll keep going, but I forget I'm already more or less at zero and that by keeping going I'm taking myself into the red, as it were, rather than leaving enough balance to get home or to cook or whatever it is I need to do next. (Sarah)

In Chapter 2 we briefly discussed illness intrusiveness. Just to remind you what this is, it refers to when an illness makes it difficult to carry out certain activities or maintain relationships – it intrudes into important aspects of your life, hence 'illness intrusiveness'. The Chronic Illness Research Team – of which I am a member – at the University of East London has looked at illness intrusiveness in a number of illnesses, including CFS/ME, IBS and Ménière's disease. Other researchers have looked at additional illnesses, such as epilepsy, HIV, lung cancer, rheumatoid arthritis and anxiety disorders. When all the results of these studies were compared, CFS/ME had the highest level of illness intrusiveness, which means that this condition impacts on different areas of life even more than an illness such as HIV. We have considered why this should be the case and think it might be because CFS/ME typically intrudes upon every area of a person's life – such as work, relationships and hobbies. We have also found that people with CFS/ME report high levels of stigma, similar to the studies by Norma Ware outlined in Chapter 3. When a person doesn't look ill it can be hard for others, including family and friends, to understand what she or he is going through. Also, because the symptoms of CFS/ME are those most people may have at some point in their lives (although not all at the same time and as severe as they can be with CFS/ME), outsiders may not appreciate the difficulties people with CFS/ME go through on a daily basis. So even though CFS/ME may not be a life-endangering illness such as HIV and lung cancer, it is still very intrusive upon people's lives and can be incredibly hard for other people to understand at a time when help is needed most.

Wired fatigue

Wired fatigue is sometimes called 'wired but tired'. This is a very frustrating symptom – you feel exhausted but your brain and nervous system seem to be on overdrive, so that you can't sleep or even rest. Wired fatigue may be linked to the hypothalamic–pituitary–adrenal (HPA) axis dysfunction that we explored in Chapter 4. If we recall, the HPA axis controls a number of hormones such as adrenaline and cortisol. Our bodies are, at times, pumped full of these hormones so that we are primed and ready for action (as in the example of chasing or fleeing from the lion). In healthy people, once a threat is gone the parasympathetic nervous system, which counteracts the processes involved in the alarm response, will kick in and readjust our hormone levels, but if there are problems with our HPA axis and its communication systems, this may not occur. At present there is very little research on wired fatigue but it is something my research group at the University of East London is interested in exploring further.

Brain fog

Brain fog is a common expression and refers to problems with cognitive function that many people with CFS/ME experience. Examples of brain fog are forgetting words, words being on the tip of your tongue but not quite reachable, difficulty in understanding things – such as following a simple plot on television, and not being able to do easy sums that you would have done with no trouble in the past, for example working out change. Here is Sarah's description of brain fog:

> It's concentration, memory, finding the right words – that sort of thing. Just feeling kind of slow in the head to pull out the words or to put the sentences together. (Sarah)

Brain fog can also be described as feeling that your head is full of treacle or that there is a curtain over your brain – you know you're still as intelligent as you were before having CFS/ME but there seems to be some kind of wall blocking out your brain's ability to function. Gerald describes his brain fog as a 'muzzy head':

> One thing a lot of people get is the muzzy head. I haven't had much muzzy head of late, which is very good because it does mean you can get on and do things better. I have had quite long periods of muzzy head though, especially when I was working full-time. I'd be going into work the whole week and really living on autopilot – getting on with my work but just wishing the day would come to an end. (Gerald)

In our research group's work we have found that after people perform cognitive tasks they frequently say that brain fog starts. However, this is a tricky symptom for researchers to capture because if people with CFS/ME are having a bad day in terms of fatigue and brain fog, they may postpone their testing session – and quite rightly so. This may be the reason why many cognitive studies of CFS/ME state that those with the condition perform as well as healthy people. Our group is devising studies to tap into the different types of fatigue so that other scientists and doctors can understand the experience of people with CFS/ME. We hope this work will help the wider scientific community and the general public to see that even though people with CFS/ME may not look ill, their symptoms are very real and impact on many, if not all, areas of life.

Flu-like fatigue

Flu-like fatigue is again very often reported by people who have CFS/ME and appears particular to this condition. This type of fatigue seems to be associated with a viral or bacterial infection, and often people report low-grade fever:

> I had a tingling – the sort of thing you expect to get better after a couple of days – and I waited and it just wouldn't go away. I'd get better for a few days and then it would just come on me again. I'd go to work in the morning and feel all right, by lunchtime my throat would be getting sore and by the time I went home I'd be aching and start running a fever. It was just like a very common sort of viral infection that just kept repeating and wouldn't go away. I went to see my GP and had a couple of courses of antibiotics – but I just could not get it to go away. (Caroline)

Some researchers believe that people with CFS/ME have viruses that are continually reactivated. Dr Amolak Bansal, an immunologist from St Helier Hospital in Surrey, who is also a member of the Chronic Illness Research Team at the University of East London, has suggested that people who have CFS/ME may be experiencing an interplay between viral infections, stress and sleep dysfunction. As we saw in Chapter 4, stress can have a significant impact on the immune system. Lack of sleep can also dampen immunity in people, meaning that the immune system is less effective in dealing with things such as viral infections. In turn, viral or bacterial infections can also put pressure on the immune system, leading to dysfunction. Stress may also be a factor involved in immune dysfunction, or both stress *and* an infection may occur at the same time. This cycle needn't be sequential –

stress may lead to sleep disturbance or vice versa, which may then make it more likely that you succumb to an infection. But of course having a nasty bug can lead to lack of sleep and stress if, for instance, you are not able to work or look after the children. If we think again about our hypothetical example of Maggie in Chapter 4, who has a demanding home and work life and then contracts glandular fever, we can see that infections rarely occur in a bubble. Most of us will have some sort of stress in our lives at most points throughout life, but infections certainly don't care about that! This theory of CFS/ME is much like the psychoneuroimmunology model of CFS/ME but differs in the assertion that stress – and/or poor sleep – can essentially reactivate the virus by dampening our immune response, resulting in flu-like symptoms again. This process then acts as a loop because the flu-like symptoms will make it hard for us to maintain our activities and roles (such as look after the kids and go to work), which leads to stress, which in turn has an impact on our immune systems.

Immune-type symptoms

In addition to the flu-like fatigue above, there are other immune-type symptoms reported by those who have CFS/ME. Here Gerald talks about his permanent sore throat – a common symptom in CFS/ME:

> Something I've observed over the years is that I always have a sore throat – 24 hours a day, 365 days a year. Now I live with it – it's so persistent I hardly notice it.

Immune-type symptoms do not only include tender lymph nodes, recurrent sore throat, recurrent flu-like symptoms but also new sensitivities to food, medications and/or chemicals – as stated in the Canadian criteria of CFS/ME (see Chapter 2). Sarah describes her severe reaction to strong smells and chemicals:

> I've got this clinical problem with perfumes and any kind of strong smelling fragrance – cooking, petrol, environmental smells – which restricts some of the things I can do or who I can be with. It's that kind of intolerance that increases dramatically if someone suddenly comes near me with something like a strong perfume – my brain will just slow down completely, my throat can hurt, my chest can hurt so that makes me sort of run away almost. I have to open the windows, which you can't always do – depends on where you are. So I have to monitor who I have here strictly, and what they do and how they come, so I have to request people to be very careful about what they put on. Even soap

powder in the clothes is another one – when people's bodies get hot the clothes give off the smell of the washing powder, so in some places, if I know people are doing those things I just can't go, and if they're not willing to cooperate – and sometimes people won't because they don't see why they should help – it is hard. So I don't do a lot in public. I go to the library but I have to be very careful even there – I have to find a place that's the least smelly: I walk past people before I decide where I'll sit. I use the computer there so I take a towel for sitting on the seat because people wear other things and it leaves a smell on the seat and it gets on my clothes; I wear a glove for using the mouse because of hand-cream on the mouse. (Sarah)

So we can see just how restrictive some of these immune-type symptoms can be. Some people with CFS/ME also appear to have numerous allergies before they become ill with CFS/ME. Researchers at the Departments of Medicine and Paediatrics within the University of Colorado Health Sciences Center in Denver looked at people with CFS/ME, people with CFS/ME and allergies, healthy people and healthy people with allergies. The research team concluded that in people with CFS/ME and allergies, allergic inflammation may have a role in the development of CFS/ME, possibly due to immune activation. This is interesting because if people with CFS/ME and allergies are indeed subtly different from those without allergies, different types of treatments could be created based on autoimmunity – allergies are an auto-immune reaction, meaning that the immune system is activated in the face of innocuous threats such as dust and pollen.

Pain

Many people with CFS/ME have pain. This can be felt in the muscles and/or joints and is often widespread. It can also seem to move around the body. Gerald describes it thus:

In fact the muscle pains in my legs were very pronounced. I'd only ever experienced these sorts of muscle pains when I'd had flu – proper flu: I don't just mean a cold, but a flu when you're in bed for a week. So I knew about these muscle pains, which feel like the beginning of cramp, but I had them quite severely. (Gerald)

Many also have quite severe headaches that seem to be new in terms of their pattern or severity as compared to before onset of CFS/ME. As mentioned in Chapter 2, there is an overlap between CFS/ME and the condition fibromyalgia. As this chapter is about symptoms and diagnosis, it might be useful to describe the differences between the two conditions so that when you visit your doctor you'll have this know-ledge at hand. People with fibromyalgia often have chronic and severe fatigue but not always. Conversely people with CFS/ME may have pain but again not always. But to be diagnosed with fibromyalgia you would have to report pain and it would need to be at specific points in the body. These are often called 'tender points'. These tender points can be very sensitive and will hurt when pressed with a finger, so much so that the patient will often flinch or jump back when the area is pressed. To be diagnosed with fibromyalgia, 11 out of 18 tender points need to be painful when pressed. These points are located throughout the body – on the neck, back, chest, elbows, hips, buttocks and knees. If you think you may have fibromyalgia rather than CFS/ME, do discuss it with your doctor because the treatments for the two disorders differ somewhat.

Sleep disturbance

When you have CFS/ME you may sleep for many hours but not feel at all better or less tired. This is known as 'unrefreshing sleep' and is also a key symptom of CFS/ME. Surprisingly perhaps, it is relatively rare to be referred to a sleep specialist if you tell your doctor you are chronically fatigued, but research has shown that people with CFS/ME often have primary sleep conditions, some of which are treat-able. In a study published 20 years ago a group of researchers based in the Department of Neurology within the State University of New York looked at sleep in 72 people with CFS/ME, 57 multiple sclerosis patients who said they had fatigue as one of their predominant symp-toms and 40 healthy people. Those with CFS/ME reported more sleep disturbance than both those with fatigue-type multiple sclerosis and those without long-term conditions. However, it was the next phase of this research that was really telling: 16 people with CFS/ME who had stated that they had poor sleep went on to have their sleep tested objectively with polysomnography. Polysomnography uses a range of measures to assess brain activity: muscle tone, airflow from the nose and mouth, heart rate and movement in the chest and abdomen. This type of test is used to diagnose sleep disorders and often requires an overnight stay at a specialist sleep centre. The polysomnography read-ings taken in the 16 people with CFS/ME in the study showed that 63 per cent of the group had clinical sleep problems, including peri-odic movement disorder (often called 'restless-leg syndrome'), sleep apnoea (where people can stop breathing in the night) and narcolepsy (where a person suddenly falls asleep at inappropriate times).

Further work on sleep in CFS/ME has recently been carried out by a group of researchers in the UK at the Northumbria Centre for Sleep Research, and the Fatigue Service at Lelystad in the Netherlands. This study found that 30 per cent of people with CFS/ME who were referred to a specialist fatigue clinic actually had a primary sleep disorder. Both this study and the study in the previous paragraph are important because they lead us to question the accuracy of CFS/ME diagnoses (we will explore misdiagnosis later in this chapter). Also, the treatment for sleep disorders is very different from those for CFS/ME, so it is vital that the correct diagnosis is made – many sleep disorders can be successfully treated so that people can return to their everyday lives.

Diagnosis

The most important thing to do when you have a long-term condition is to get the correct diagnosis. This may not always be an easy task because the symptoms of CFS/ME are very similar to those of many other illnesses. As mentioned in the introduction to this chapter, a diagnosis can be difficult to obtain, but the situation does seem to be getting better as newly qualified doctors are – sometimes – trained in conditions such as CFS/ME. Sadly, this does not mean a great deal of time is spent on the condition in medical school, but at least it's mentioned and a number of the local support groups in the UK have been giving talks to medical students so that they can understand what it's like to have CFS/ME. Here Linda Webb, the former chairperson of the Richmond and Kingston ME Group, explains how the group has been trying to influence medical training:

> Members of Richmond and Kingston ME Group have been talking to medical students from St George's Hospital Tooting over the last few years under the auspices of Integrated Neurological Services, a Twickenham-based charity. We talk on a one-to-one basis or to a small group of students about the symptoms, living with ME, its potential severity, how we got a diagnosis, and the effect ME has had on our careers, families and friends. We have all found this a positive experience as the students are enthusiastic and want to know more about the illness. For people with ME who have been disbelieved by their GPs or consultants, someone who listens to them is like finding gold dust. In the long run we hope that a new generation of GPs and consultants will have a basic understanding of this neurological condition when they meet people with ME in their medical practice. (Linda Webb)

But despite local groups' activities, many people do still report difficult experiences in gaining a diagnosis:

> I went back to my GP and I said: 'I've got earache. Can you look at my ears?', and I explained all these other symptoms. I said: 'In the mornings I just feel too tired to get up and go to work', and she said: 'Oh, I think maybe you've got depression', and I said: 'Well, what about the earache?' It was strange, so I didn't get any kind of help there. (Emma)

Other people have said that their GPs thought they had depression. This is perhaps an easy – but unacceptable – mistake to make because depression and CFS/ME can appear very similar on the surface. This is why it is important to write down your symptoms and take the list with you when you go – all too often it is impossible to remember everything when there is a packed waiting room and the bright lighting has made you feel much worse, not to mention actually having to get to the GP practice in the first place. So take a list or even better a short diary of your symptoms – this will help the GP to diagnose you accurately.

Your doctor will need to rule out any other causes of the symptoms before coming to a diagnosis of CFS/ME; therefore she or he will order a number of blood tests. The standard tests are those recommended by the National Institute for Health and Care Excellence (NICE is the body that sets out detailed guidance for doctors in the UK). The NICE guidelines for CFS/ME are as shown in Table 1.

Table 1 The NICE testing guidelines for CFS/ME

Test	Indicative of
urinalysis for protein, blood and glucose	kidney function and diabetes
full blood count	anaemia, cancers
liver function	liver disorders
thyroid function	over or underactive thyroid
erythrocyte sedimentation rate or plasma viscosity	general illness/inflammation
C-reactive protein	general illness/inflammation
random blood glucose	diabetes
serum creatinine	kidney function
screening blood tests	for gluten sensitivity/coeliac disease
serum calcium	disorders of calcium
creatine kinase	muscle disorders
assessment of serum ferritin levels (children and young people only)	anaemia or haemochromatosis

If these tests come back negative and there are no other clinical signs or features of another disorder, the doctor will consider a diagnosis of CFS/ME. However, this again is not always a clear path:

> When I went back in to get the results they asked me: 'Did you think it was cancer?', and I thought: 'No, I never even thought it was cancer.' I said: 'Is it ME? Could it be ME?' and they said: 'Well, we don't know what to do with it. We don't call it ME.' And that was it. (Lucy)

Fortunately not everyone has a difficult time with their doctors. Gerald rather amusingly says that this may be to do with his gender, but I assure you this is not always the case.

> My doctor was very understanding. I'd been very lucky with him, but then you see I'm tall, I'm male, I'm articulate – I advise ME sufferers not to be short, female and inarticulate: doctors treat them with disdain. (Gerald)

Once your doctor has diagnosed CFS/ME there are a number of treatment options and self-management strategies (see Chapters 6–9).

Misdiagnosis

Unfortunately misdiagnoses can occur, even with doctors' best intentions. In a study carried out in Newcastle and published in 2010, investigators looked at the medical notes of people who were diagnosed with CFS/ME. The rates of misdiagnosis were quite shocking. Of the 260 case notes examined, 40 per cent of the referrals to the Newcastle NHS Chronic Fatigue Syndrome Service should not have been diagnosed with CFS/ME. Of those misdiagnosed, 47 per cent were found to have another disorder that could explain their symptoms. Examples of the types of illnesses people were subsequently diagnosed with included metabolic syndrome (8 cases), neurological disorder (13 cases), connective tissue disorder or autoimmune disease (9 cases) and issues such as low body mass index, haemochromatosis (a genetic disorder), microprolactinoma (an endocrine condition) and Lyme disease (all of which accounted for one case each). Of those initially misdiagnosed, 20 per cent actually had primary sleep disorders such as sleep apnoea – a potentially life-threatening disorder in which people stop breathing for short periods of time – and restless-leg syndrome. Psychological or psychiatric conditions accounted for 15 per cent of misdiagnoses, and 4 per cent in fact had a cardiovascular illness. Idiopathic fatigue, whereby there is seemingly no medical explanation for the fatiguing symptoms, was documented for 13 per cent of referrals. Many of these illnesses have their own treatment strategies, so it is very important for patients to get the right diagnosis so that they can access the correct treatments and see a relevant specialist. Also, the researchers in this study suggested that it might be better for health services to focus on symptoms rather than the underlying disease process, as this would allow people with numerous types of fatiguing conditions to attend specialist fatigue clinics – in the UK where this study was carried out, only those with a diagnosis of CFS/ME are able to receive treatment at this type of clinic. The issue of misdiagnosis in people who present with chronic fatigue does seem to be a common problem – another study based in London and carried out in 2012 found that almost half – 49 per cent – of referrals to a specialist CFS/ME service were of people who had other conditions.

Summary and conclusion

This chapter has looked in more detail at some of the key symptoms in CFS/ME, with case studies added to help us understand the lived experience of the condition. The tests a doctor will do if he or she thinks you have CFS/ME were also outlined. Finally the important issue of misdiagnosis was outlined because recent research has shown that a high proportion of people with CFS/ME may have other conditions that would explain their symptoms. In the next chapter we will begin to explore the treatment options available if you have been diagnosed with CFS/ME.

6

On the road to recovery:
orthodox treatments

In this chapter we will look at some mainstream treatments that your doctor may suggest you try. These include psychobehavioural techniques and also some medicines that can be prescribed to help with certain symptoms. The treatments in this chapter are options that you can access through your GP, although for the psychobehavioural approaches you will need a referral to a clinical psychologist or physiotherapist.

> As it happens, my NHS consultant told me on the first visit that he didn't have any test results back yet. It wasn't like he knew I was a special subject, he just looked me in the eye and told me I would get better. He said it might take a while but I would, and I'm eternally grateful to him for that. (Mary)

It is important to know that your health can improve. It may take time to find the right treatment for you because everyone with CFS/ME has a different profile of symptoms. Therefore the first step is gaining a collaborative relationship with your doctor. As mentioned in the previous chapter, CFS/ME is not often taught comprehensively – if at all – in medical schools. You may feel you know more about your condition than your doctor, and this could well be true. So following diagnosis, it can be important to work with the myriad symptoms with your doctor and appreciate that at this time there is no one-size-fits-all treatment for everyone with CFS/ME. In time, when further research has been carried out and we start to understand more about the precise nature of the mechanisms underlying the condition, it may be easier to tailor treatments to individuals. We will look at the future of treatment in Chapter 10, but for now let's explore what's on offer at the moment.

Medications for symptom management

In terms of managing specific symptoms, your doctor may want to prescribe certain drugs that can help with problems such as pain and poor sleep. Although these have not been shown in research studies to 'cure' CFS/ME, they can, for some people, offer relief of individual symptoms. However, people with CFS/ME often report being sensitive to medications, so your doctor may advise a very low dose to start with.

Your doctor may suggest you try a low-dose tricyclic antidepressant – usually one called amitriptyline – to help with sleep problems and pain. Tricyclic antidepressants are one of the oldest types of antidepressant, and work by influencing chemicals in our brains called neurotransmitters. Neurotransmitters have many different roles, including controlling and regulating bodily functions. Noradrenaline and serotonin are two neurotransmitters that regulate our mood, and tricyclic antidepressants work by preventing the reabsorption of these substances into nerve cells. As noradrenaline and serotonin are mood enhancers, by impeding their reabsorption, their positive effects can be maintained. It is not fully clear why they appear to help with pain and sleep disturbance, but research does show that in low doses, tricyclic antidepressants can help with pain and poor sleep in those with CFS/ME. However, do discuss this with your doctor if you are currently taking any other form of antidepressant, in particular selective serotonin reuptake inhibitors – taking both at the same time may lead to adverse interactions.

As noted, antidepressants can also help with low mood and symptoms of anxiety and depression. If you have these symptoms please do not be reluctant to talk them through with your doctor. Having a chronic illness can be very distressing, so it is perfectly reasonable to seek help for all of your symptoms, not just the fatigue and pain. However, as some researchers and medics have noted, while these medicines can lift mood and help if someone is very anxious, they will probably not reduce the fatigue and other symptoms you may have – for example, cognitive difficulties such as problems with memory and concentration, and autonomic disturbances such as cold feet and hands. So it is important to be realistic about the scope of these drugs – false promises followed by disappointment certainly don't make anyone feel better.

The substance melatonin is sometimes recommended for children and young adults with CFS/ME but not for older adults. This may be due to the conflicting evidence regarding the treatment: some studies have shown that people improved in terms of fatigue, concentration, motivation and activity, whereas others did not find these effects. Melatonin is a hormone that is secreted by the endocrine system, and it also acts as a neurotransmitter. Its function is to help regulate the sleep–wake cycle (also known as the circadian rhythm), hence it is sometimes prescribed for insomnia. Melatonin can be purchased from high-street natural health stores, but do talk to your doctor if you're interested in it as the research remains inconclusive in CFS/ME.

Even though many people with CFS/ME state that they first became ill with a virus or bacterial infection, treatments based on antiviral and antibacterial medications have not shown promise. It is not clear why there are anecdotal reports of improvements with antibiotics and anti-virals – it may be because individuals were misdiagnosed and actually had some other sort of infection, such as Lyme disease. Be that as it may, there is not currently enough evidence for the use of these types of medicines in CFS/ME.

Similarly hormonal treatments – such as hydrocortisone and thy-roxine – do not have enough evidence of effectiveness behind them to be routinely used in CFS/ME, even though some studies have shown hormonal irregularities in those with the condition (for example, low cortisol levels). All medications carry risks and have side effects, so at the present time, unless your blood tests show deficiencies in specific hormones, it is unlikely hormonal treatments would be prescribed. In the same vein, even though we have discussed various immunological abnormalities in those with CFS/ME, there is no definitive data to suggest that immunotherapy is beneficial in its treatment.

Non-pharmacological (psychobehavioural) treatments

The doctor said: 'Believe me, I know what's wrong with you. You don't need to do anything at all. Just go home and put your feet up. That's it – end of story, because you're signed off for the rest of your life.' And that was that really. Even he didn't realize at the time how bad some of my symptoms were, and it actually took about eight years to cover all the ground that needed to be covered. I'm still not convinced that everything is being covered, that I couldn't do more. (Deborah)

Although Deborah's doctor was very supportive and kind to tell her to 'put her feet up', most of us want to have active lives. This is why people with CFS/ME can often go through 'boom-and-bust' patterns, whereby when symptoms are at a minimum they try to do all the things that were impossible when symptom levels were high, such as laundry that has built up, other housework, catching up with friends and so on – an activity boom in other words (see Figure 1). This often then leads, unsurprisingly, to an activity bust and an exacerbation of fatigue and other symptoms. It can be incredibly difficult to get out of this pattern because chronic illness can create a great deal of guilt surrounding not being able to do what we did previously. However, as a long-term strategy, boom-and-bust is very detrimental and can make people increasingly unwell. Behavioural treatments aim to overcome this pattern in order to assist recovery.

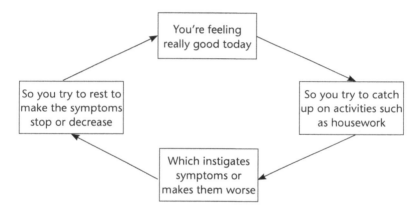

Figure 1 Boom and bust in CFS/ME

Cognitive behavioural therapy

The theory behind cognitive behavioural therapy (CBT) is that it works on the basis that psychological and social factors (such as, respectively, personality type or traits and stressful working environment) inter-act with physiological processes (such as raised or decreased cortisol output), hence this treatment is aligned with the biopsychosocial model we discussed in Chapter 3. CBT is most often conducted by a clinical psychologist, health psychologist or CBT therapist specifically trained in this technique – that is, it would be unusual for your GP or a specialist medical doctor to carry out the treatment. But this is not to say that CBT is only for people with psychological problems – it is used to help cope with many different conditions, including rheumatoid arthritis, chronic pain and insomnia. In the session the CBT therapist or psychologist will work with patients on their 'cognitions' – how people think about certain situations and the beliefs that they hold. This is based on the theory that negative thought patterns and beliefs can lead to disadvantageous coping behaviours, which in turn can heighten symptoms. So if we take the issue of activity boom-and-bust in CFS/ME, a negative thought pattern may be: 'I need to catch up on all the washing and ring my family and make the dinner, otherwise I'm just a useless person', which will lead someone to try to do all these things when she simply does not have enough gas in the tank. CBT can help us to reappraise the situation and know that we are not useless if we can't do all the housework. This can then allow us to focus on one activity at a time – for instance phoning family members – and help us to believe that doing that one thing is enough when we are unwell. To assist with this the therapist and patient will work through a number of exercises, often including 'homework' for the patient to do and practise outside of the session. This homework can also help reduce rumination, worry and anxiety (we will talk more about rumination in the next chapter, along with other ways to break recurring thought patterns). This is the 'cognitive' bit in CBT, and the theory states that once this is altered, more constructive behaviour will emerge.

CBT is one of the most researched treatments for CFS/ME, possibly because psychiatrists became interested in this condition after the publication of McEvedy's and Beard's paper in the *British Medical Journal* (as discussed in Chapter 1). There have been meta-analyses of CBT for the treatment of CFS/ME. A meta-analysis is a review of all the studies carried out on a topic, with some complicated statistics thrown in to try to get an overall picture of whether a treatment works. These types of analyses are seen to be very convincing as they can aggregate much larger bodies of data than would be possible in any one research study. In this example by researchers based at the University of Oxford and led by the senior researcher Jonathan Price, 15 studies with a total of 1,043 people with CFS/ME were combined together. When CBT was compared with usual care (that is, the help and advice you would receive from your GP), those in the CBT groups showed better responses to the treatment: 40 per cent of people undergoing CBT had lower fatigue scores as compared to 26 per cent of those in the usual care group. When CBT was compared to other types of psychological therapies such as counselling, relaxation and support, those who received CBT sessions also had better overall improvements in levels of fatigue.

However, as with most research these findings do need to be viewed with some caution. When the researchers looked at the people's fatigue in the longer term (1–7 months after treatment finished), and included the information from people who did not finish the treatment, there was no difference in fatigue levels between the CBT group and the group who received usual care. Also, the studies in this review tended not to look at how acceptable the treatment was to the people in the research (that is, whether they felt CBT was an appropriate technique for the condition), which can be an important aspect of whether someone will finish a treatment, and of course if they will take it up in the first place.

CBT and graded exercise therapy (which we will move on to next) aren't viewed as being acceptable by some people. Some researchers and medics have theorized that the core issue in CFS/ME is psychological in nature, hence a psychological therapy is the best course of action. As we explored in Chapter 3, the body and mind interact and so there is undoubtedly a psychological aspect to most, if not all, illnesses. However, the insistence that CFS/ME is *only* a psychological disorder is unacceptable to many people, and as we have seen from Chapters 3 and 4, this assertion is plainly false. As we come to understand more and more about the pathways that link the body and the mind, it seems feasible that a psychological therapy could help with some aspects of numerous illnesses, not just CFS/ME. This may explain why CBT has been shown in research studies to help symptoms of people with CFS/ME.

I had a few sessions of CBT with a private hypnotherapist in the first year of my illness. The first CBT session was about my perfectionism. I hadn't personally regarded myself as a perfectionist, but the therapist thought it was a contributing factor to my illness. I certainly believed that if you are going to do something, then you might just as well do it as well as you can and, according to the therapist, this belief made me push myself too hard beyond what my body can cope with. So perhaps I was a perfectionist after all, and it was a good session to have – but it didn't have any effect on my fatigue and I still like to do things well. This was in the beginning of my illness, which continued to get worse. After a few sessions I was no longer well enough to travel to the therapist, so I had to stop. But I don't believe it was the therapy that made me worse – it just wasn't effective enough to make me better. I am still very driven and definitely an over-doer, so I have the tendency to push myself too hard because I can get very enthusiastic about things and find it difficult to stop on time before I completely collapse. Psychologically, then, perhaps there's still work to be done. (Hayley)

Graded exercise therapy (GET)

GET is a technique whereby activity is gradually increased over time in an effort to improve a person's functioning and reduce the symptoms of CFS/ME. This type of treatment is often used in physiotherapy and rehabilitation programmes and has been adapted for use in CFS/ME. GET starts with a physical assessment so that a 'baseline' of activity can be met, where symptoms do not immediately get worse. Then there will be a discussion between the physiotherapist or specialist GET practitioner and the patient so that appropriate goals can be set – for example, walking to the post office, cleaning a room, meeting a friend for lunch. There will be a number of steps to reach this goal, each increasing in intensity until the goal is met.

GET has also been looked at in a meta-analysis, this time by researchers based in London and again with Jonathan Price of the University of Oxford. There were fewer studies in this analysis than the CBT review – only five published studies could be included. The review found that people receiving GET were less fatigued than those just under usual care – their normal doctor's care – and also less fatigued than people who were prescribed antidepressants. Interestingly, people who participated in combined approaches where GET was offered alongside patient education were less fatigued at 12 weeks than those on the single-therapy programme. However, dropout rates were high in the GET groups, which may suggest that individuals with CFS/ME are averse to this type of therapy or even that these people felt GET was making their condition worse.

These high dropout rates, or numbers of people who did not finish the GET programmes, are important to think about when considering therapies. The ME Association – a UK-based charity for people with ME and CFS/ME – carried out an online survey that asked questions about the treatments its members had tried. Of the 906 respondents to the questions about GET, 33 per cent said they were 'much worse' after the treatment (23 per cent said they felt slightly worse, 21 per cent reported no change in symptoms, 19 per cent improved and 3 per cent had improved greatly). Similarly, Action for ME – AfME, the second main UK-based ME and CFS/ME charity – found that 60 per cent of respondents in their survey said GET had made their condition worse, of whom 44 per cent reported much or very much worse symptom levels. In terms of improvement, 22 per cent of people in the AfME survey reported improvement following GET. This information of course should also be viewed with caution as surveys can be biased – perhaps people who had a hard time with GET were more likely to respond than people who had recovered somewhat – but it is useful when trying to understand why some people dropped out of the trial. Finally, it should be noted that a recent large-scale study known as the PACE trial – which compared pacing (which we will discuss in the next chapter), CBT, GET and specialist medical care – reported that GET was a safe treatment for CFS/ME. However, this piece of research is a hotly debated topic, perhaps because of stories like Hayley's:

> This year I was asked to participate in a GET trial by a specialist hospital clinic. Because in recent years I have been slightly better, I thought perhaps I should try it again to see if it makes any difference. The researchers' opinion was that I had previously gone downhill as a result of GET because the initial baseline had been too high. So this time we were super-careful to make sure it was done sensitively. Initially, while I was close to my baseline there didn't seem to be any harm but there was no benefit either. But once the exercise levels were increased, I noticed I was beginning to struggle. I was able to do my exercises as prescribed, but I was no longer able to do anything in the garden and I was beginning to struggle with cooking. This was around October time, and I typically go downhill in the autumn, so it could have been just a seasonal pattern. But the exercise certainly wasn't helping me get over that pattern. In the end I was getting quite low because I was feeling so unwell that once the trial was over, I abandoned the exercise programme. I still do gentle yoga and make sure I go on mini-walks twice a day, but I'm doing it in a much more relaxed way and not five times a week. (Hayley)

In addition to negative experiences of GET, some people would prefer not to engage in this approach because it is based in part on the 'deconditioning theory' of CFS/ME. This theory states that when a person's muscles are no longer used due to a period of ill health, they become deconditioned; therefore the way to reduce symptoms is to get the muscles in working order again. However, there is an increasing amount of evidence that the muscle weakness associated with CFS/ME is actually caused by abnormalities in the muscles themselves rather than deconditioning. This could be why for some people GET seems to worsen CFS/ME rather than improve it.

One final thought on GET is that the key to this therapy is that it asks people to increase activity in a planned, sequential way. This may prove difficult for some people because if they cannot reach the goal set, it can lead to disappointment and a further sense of loss in a condition where losses can already be great. This differs from the 'pacing' technique discussed in the next chapter, which has a more flexible approach. However, research studies have shown that CBT and GET *can* be helpful for people with CFS/ME:

> When we get ME we lose control of many aspects of our lives. One way some of us try to manage this situation is by taking complete charge of tried treatments – to the extent of dismissing ones that might help. Not many are offered by medical professionals. CBT and GET can in fact get you back in to life. Taken very slowly and used consistently, they have worked for me. The time came when I stopped worrying whether I would be tarred with the 'psychological' label and simply benefited from what was on offer. (Chloe)

Summary and conclusion

This chapter has looked at some medications that are, and are not, used for symptomatic treatment in CFS/ME. Following this we explored two of the most widely recommended psychobehavioural therapies for CFS/ME: CBT and GET. Sadly none of these treatments is a 'cure' for CFS/ME, but there is a body of evidence that they can be beneficial in some people. You may therefore want to discuss these options with your healthcare practitioner, such as your psychologist, physiotherapist or GP. In the next chapter we will explore an approach called pacing that many people have said helps with CFS/ME.

7

One step at a time: pacing

In the previous chapter we discussed a number of treatment options that should be accessible through your GP or specialist practitioner. In this chapter we will outline a therapy called 'pacing' that you can try at home. Although there haven't been as many research studies investigating this technique as there have been for cognitive behavioural therapy (CBT) and graded exercise therapy (GET), many people who have tried pacing have found it to be helpful, so it may be something you could consider.

As we discovered in Chapter 6, many people reported in the ME Association and Action for ME (AfME) surveys that CBT and GET were unhelpful. However, 82 per cent of the AfME survey's respondents stated that they found pacing helpful. Pacing, also known as 'adaptive pacing therapy', is another type of activity management that attempts to break the boom-and-bust pattern we discussed in the previous chapter, and it is one you can do on your own. Nearly 60 per cent of those who completed the ME Association survey said they improved following pacing, and 12 per cent responded that they had 'greatly improved'. The main difference between pacing and GET is that the former balances activities with rest periods while the latter is more focused on sequential increases in activity. Furthermore, when pacing, activities are increased when someone is able whereas during a programme of GET the regime may be less flexible (although in practice an experienced physiotherapist advising GET may indeed suggest a flexible approach).

Like GET, the first step in a pacing programme is to establish a baseline of activities. Your baseline is how much activity you can do before becoming symptomatic or before symptoms worsen. A symptom and activity diary can help you determine what your baseline is – you may have already started one to help your doctor with your diagnosis. AfME provides a good example from the Frenchay Hospital, Bristol, in its booklet *Pacing for People with ME*, which can be downloaded from the AfME website – see Useful addresses at the end of this book. In this diary each day is divided into hour slots; to fill the diary out there is a colour coding scheme with different colours representing sleep, rest, low demand activity, medium demand activity and high demand activity. If your symptoms are very severe, particularly cognitive symptoms, do ask a member of your family or a friend to help you complete the diary. If you don't have anyone to help you, it's not necessary to use such a diary – you can simply note down your activities and your symptoms on paper or in a journal.

When filling out a diary, do remember that not all activities are 'active' per se. Activities can be emotionally and mentally demanding, not just physically demanding. For instance, you may have an elderly aunt whom you call every other day to see how she is. This may be exhausting for you as she is partly deaf, so you need to repeat yourself over and over again. She may also make you feel guilty for not visiting her more often. So although you can lie in bed and call her, this can still be incredibly draining and cause your symptoms to worsen before the call, immediately after and possibly for hours or even days after. Therefore this would be documented in your diary as a 'high demand activity'. Similarly, watching the television or reading a magazine can be mentally challenging with CFS/ME, even though other people may find this relaxing. External things that you may not have control over can also be demanding in terms of your available energy – for instance, you may live near a school and the talking/shouting children may cause you to have symptoms. This of course is not an activity but it is relevant because the noise is something you are coping with on a day-to-day basis.

Establishing a baseline

Once you have completed the diary for a few days or a week you may be surprised by how few rest and sleep periods you actually have. By looking at the relationship between your activity and symptoms you can start to get a picture of your baseline – that is, how much you can do both on a good day or a bad day before symptoms start or become worse. The next step in pacing is to reach a sustainable level of activity, and to do this you will need to stick to your baseline, even if you're having a really good day. This amount of activity may seem quite, if not very, low. This is all right so please do not be tempted to do more than you can – the purpose of establishing a baseline is to start breaking the boom-and-bust pattern. By limiting activity you're allowing your body's natural healing abilities to emerge. This takes patience and it is completely normal to have stumbles where you overdo it and your symptoms become worse again. Try not to become angry or frustrated (though of course this is difficult), rather think of this as a learning curve – you will become better at maintaining your baseline with practice.

To help you reach a point where your symptoms are stable, do use the diary to keep track of your activity but also schedule rest and relaxation periods.

Stop rules

Before moving on to ways to increase activity, it can be beneficial to know that different people have and do pace in subtly different ways. Some of these different methods can lead to setbacks, so before you start pacing do consider a number of 'stop rules'. Stop rules refers to how people know when to stop doing an activity; techniques include 'fighting it', 'listening to your body', 'using time' and 'using activity'.

'Fighting it' is when an activity has to halt because symptoms become so severe that it is impossible to carry on any longer. As you can probably imagine, it is not the most constructive type of pacing because it can lead to setbacks. When someone is actively fighting their condition they are likely to remain in the boom-and-bust pattern, which does not lead to recovery. You may find that some people with CFS/ME say that they practise this type of pacing but it is not pacing per se and is not recommended.

'Listening to your body' can be a more positive way for people to recover from CFS/ME but this approach also has drawbacks. If someone is using this stop rule then they will cease activity when symptoms increase or change. One downside of the rule is that it can become quite miserable trying to track every small increase in fatigue, pain and other symptoms, and sometimes focusing on symptoms can make them even worse. Another problem with this stop rule is linked to one of the core symptoms of CFS/ME, namely post-exertional fatigue. This type of fatigue doesn't necessarily occur straight after an activity – it can be hours or even days afterwards that the fatigue bites back. Hence 'listening to your body' would not work in this sense, so if delayed fatigue – or any other delayed symptom – is part of your CFS/ME, consider the options below instead.

The final two stop rules use your experience to guide decisions on how much activity you should do, and can be used when pacing. As such they offer more controllable ways to pace. 'Using time' as a stop rule can be a useful way to break down activities into manageable chunks, and with rest or relaxation added in, goals may be achieved. For instance, you may want to do some housework. Instead of trying to vacuum the entire house this task can be broken down into time slots. You may know that you become symptomatic after 10 minutes of vacuuming, so instead of continuing with this activity until symptoms worsen, vacuum only for five minutes. Then have a 15-minute break. You may then find you can do another five minutes of vacuuming because you have not pushed your body beyond its stop point. Using this stop rule can be a very different mind-set than you are used to because most of us like to finish a task once it's started. However, remember to be kind to yourself – this is key to preventing a boom-and-bust cycle from occurring. If you've only managed to vacuum half the house in the ten minutes over two sessions, with a rest period in between, it is all right. Pacing is a gradual process that may and probably will be frustrating, but give yourself and your body time to recover. It can be helpful to think of pacing as rehabilitation: if someone lost the use of their legs after an accident you wouldn't expect that person to get up and run a marathon the day after surgery, so don't put these high – and unrealistic – expectations on yourself.

'Using activities' is a very similar stop rule to 'using time' but here you use the amount of activity as a stopping point rather than duration. It is still based on previous experience. To give an example, you may know that reading two emails will not cause mental fatigue but trying to read everything in your inbox will definitely cause not only mental fatigue but headaches and brain fog. Therefore look at your inbox and read the two most important messages and then rest or relax before looking at another two. Screen-time may seem like an innocuous form of activity but even in people without CFS/ME, spending too much time on the computer, tablet, smartphone or watching TV can be exhausting and certainly are activities in themselves. So even though you might feel on one particularly good day that you could just quickly take a peek at a third and fourth message, stop at two emails to prevent post-exertional or delayed fatigue occurring. In time you will be able to increase the activity intervals, but during pacing do try to be strict with yourself to prevent getting back into a boom-and-bust pattern.

While 'fighting it' and 'listening to your body' may seem intuitive methods of pacing, and 'using time' and 'using activities' more contrived, there is a sound reason why the latter stop rules can be a positive aspect of your recovery programme. By using time or activities to pace, you will have a pretty good idea of how much you will be able to do before you start, even if this is a much smaller amount than you used to be able or would like to do. If you rely on the first two stop rules your symptoms will stop you doing something not only on the day but possibly later in the week, if you experience delayed fatigue. So if you use time or activities to pace, you can finish what you set out to do even if this is only a small amount, and you can feel good about yourself for that. In a sense this is taking back control rather than letting the CFS/ME control you. Finally, it can be much easier to explain your pacing programme to people if you can say 'I can do ten minutes of walking but then I need a five-minute rest before I can finish the outing', or 'It may take me longer to prepare dinner than it used to because I need to do the veg. prep, then sit down and relax, before starting the actual cooking', instead of 'I'm not sure how far I can go/if I can finish cooking this meal as it will just depend on my symptoms.'

Increasing activity

If you are using 'fighting it' or 'listening to your body' as ways to pace, the next stage of pacing may be a little tricky. It can be very difficult indeed to increase activity if you've been fighting the condition, because you'll be at your maximum capacity already. If you've been 'listening to your body' you may attend even more to your symptoms when you increase activity, which in itself may amplify sensations. This can lead to further frustration in an already exasperating illness. Increasing activity in chunks of either time or bite-sized parts of tasks are generally more productive and rewarding types of activity increase. This is also known as 'pacing-up'. If you know your baseline really well – that is, what you can manage in terms of time or activity chunks – you can make a clear decision on by how much you should 'pace-up'.

However, the general guidance from the main CFS/ME charities and patient organizations on increasing activity when pacing states that you should only increase activities by 10 per cent at a time. For instance, if you can comfortably vacuum for 10 minutes, then when you pace-up you should only attempt 11 minutes of vacuuming. This is obviously somewhat trickier when using activity to pace. Every person's recovery is different, so start slowly. Bigger increases may be achieved later in recovery – be as patient with yourself as you can.

You may be wondering when the best time to pace-up is. This again varies from person to person but the crucial barometer must be that you can confidently sustain the current level of activity on both a good *and* a bad day. When you're starting to pace, and also when you're establishing your baseline, this level of activity may seem depressingly low. But rather than viewing the current situation this way, instead see it as an investment in your future. By limiting your activities so that they are sustainable, your body will be able to recover without having to fight back in the form of giving you more severe symptoms. If you don't feel able to pace-up at a particular point (which may be because of countless issues – sadly, the world doesn't stop around us just because we've had to slow down), then don't feel the need to force yourself. This is the main difference between GET and pacing: there are no set rules as to when and how activity increase should occur. *You* have the control here, so do not feel pressed by others to pace more quickly than your body will comfortably allow.

Setbacks

Even if you are very careful with pacing you may experience a setback, especially when first trying to establish a baseline. This is completely normal: pacing is far from easy – but bear in mind it will get easier. Also, we live in environments that often put demands on us, even when we're actively trying to get well. Sometimes, even if we have tried to communicate our pacing programme to others, along with the fact that it is a gradual process, people can have expectations of us based on our capabilities before CFS/ME. Boundaries are very important here, and setting them is an activity in itself that can be 'high demand', so make sure to record these interactions in your activity diary.

You may have to start saying 'no' a lot more. This can certainly be hard both for you and the recipient, but know that it is for your future health. Not being the person to whom everyone comes in a crisis may feel like the illness is taking away part of your identity. It's not – in fact it's putting you back in control of your life. Priorities will need to be reassessed and often reset. Guilt may arise because you have to let go of some of your former roles – you should understand that you can only be there for others if you initially put yourself and your health first. These can be tough emotional and mental processes to deal with, so ask for help. If your family and friends cannot support you then peer support (such as a local CFS/ME support group) or professional care (such as a counsellor or therapist) can help. For this segment of your life, put yourself and your health on the top of the priority list. If you have dependants, gain as much practical support as you can. The one caveat is: do not give up everything that brings you joy. In fact when pacing-up, be sure to include pleasurable activities wherever possible – that way you can maintain your identity even if you can't do all the things you did before you were ill.

The importance of stages, severity and support

However, although many people with CFS/ME have said that pacing has helped them recover from CFS/ME, if you are in the very initial stage of the illness it is more important to rest and give your body a chance to deal with any infection. For example, if you had an infection a number of weeks ago that does not seem to shift, but you have not yet been diagnosed, it is definitely advisable to rest completely. As Charles Shepherd, the ME Association's medical advisor (who has also had personal experience of the condition), states:

> Finding the right balance will depend on the stage, severity and degree of fluctuation in symptoms that is being experienced. During the very early stages of an acute onset ME (i.e. within the first few weeks following a viral infection), a period of rest, possibly including a period of bed rest, is advisable. Ideally this should then be followed by a period of convalescence and (hopefully) improvement involving very gradual and flexible increases in both physical and mental activity.

This point about the stage of illness is very important but hasn't been researched yet. It is to be hoped that, in time, studies will be published looking at precisely which techniques are best used at which stage, so that there is clearer guidance. (In fact very little is known about the stages of CFS/ME, or indeed if there are any, so this is also a required area of research.)

In addition to considering the stage and severity of your CFS/ME before embarking on a pacing programme, it can also be useful to find a 'buddy' for support along the way. Pacing is taught in some specialist CFS/ME services but if you haven't had the opportunity, or health, to attend one of these it can be useful to contact your local area support group and ask if anyone else is using pacing at the moment.

> Pacing is of course not easy, even if you know how you should be doing it, so I think it would be useful, in an ideal world, to have a 'personal pacing trainer' for ongoing support. It is true that the group has a couple of follow-up meetings every few months, but these group-based meetings are probably not the right forum for discussing any personal

day-to-day difficulties with pacing. For this reason, I and another member of the group formed a little pacing support group for ourselves, so that we wouldn't forget all the advice after the programme was finished. (Chloe)

Finally, pacing, as with all current approaches to the treatment of CFS/ ME, can have drawbacks:

Pacing was a part of the local hospital programme, and after the programme I tried to implement all the pacing advice I had been taught. I tried to do it as carefully as I could, measuring my baseline for various activities, making a daily schedule and using an alarm clock to stop me from overdoing things (without an alarm clock I would never remember to stop whatever I was doing before I had completely exhausted myself). For example, one of my activities was gardening, and at the time I could manage three minutes a day, in three one-minute chunks. Another ME friend that I had met at the clinic was doing pacing with me, and we'd have regular phone calls to give each other mutual support to make sure we didn't give up. I really made an effort for about three or four months, but I was not improving at all. In fact I noticed that such a strict form of pacing made me really anxious and stressed. I found it very tedious and the method didn't really suit my personality at all. I was just constantly feeling grumpy, and really resented having to stop if I was doing something nice. So in the end, as it wasn't doing any good, I gave up. Having said that, I do know I go downhill if I overdo things, so these days I naturally pace myself in a more relaxed way, without a clock. My pacing friend was much better at being self-disciplined about pacing, and she is in fact much better now. All in all I would say pacing is a necessary part of a life with ME – you just need to find the level of strictness that you personally can live with. (Hayley)

Summary and conclusion

In this chapter we have looked at an approach called pacing that many people have said has helped them with their CFS/ME. You can try this yourself at home but, as noted above, it can be useful to have a pacing buddy to compare notes and help deal with the difficulties of a pacing programme and setbacks. In the next chapter we will describe some of the most common alternative and complementary techniques that have been used by people with CFS/ME, and in Chapter 9 there will be a discussion of various things you can do yourself to manage symptoms.

8

Supplements and complementary and alternative therapies

In the previous two chapters we explored a number of approaches for tackling CFS/ME based on psychological, behavioural and activity-management strategies, as well as some medicines that may be prescribed for specific symptoms. These are the treatments that are most widely available through your GP or specialist practitioner but they are not by any means the only therapies there are. In this chapter we will outline just some of the less mainstream approaches, often called 'complementary and alternative medicine' (CAM). The focus here is on the most common CAM treatments people with CFS/ME try, but the list is not exhaustive – that would require another book!

> There are so many different things people will tell you. If you don't understand what the illness is, you'll find that you'll read in the paper something saying that this or that is the way to go about it – changing diet and changing this, that and the other. You change various bits and parts of your life but there are 1,001 things that you get in terms of advice, and in terms of trying to work out what are the two or three things that might be very useful. It takes a long time to sort all that out. When I was first ill it was colonic irrigation and that sort of thing – very fashionable in those days, not that I ever tried but it could have been a way forward for me. (Peter)

In addition to all the advice you may receive from well-meaning family, friends and acquaintances, the web is awash with information and misinformation. A study published in 2002 that reviewed 225 websites – so only a small proportion – found that 80 per cent contained inaccuracies regarding CFS/ME research. So do be cautious when reading claims made online. Also, it is worth bearing in mind that government agencies such as the National Institute for Health and Care Excellence (NICE), which reviews published research relating to the effectiveness of specific treatments for diagnosable health conditions in the UK, do not advocate CAM treatments for CFS/ME at the moment. This is likely to change when more research studies are conducted and published about CAM for the treatment of CFS/ME. Nevertheless many approaches are used by people with CFS/ME. As this area is not as comprehensively regulated as traditional medicine – that is, there are fewer safety nets and avenues for recourse if you have a negative experience – there is some advice about finding a reputable CAM practitioner at the end of the chapter.

Supplements

Every day we are bombarded with advice on diet, and often there are news stories advising that we need more of vitamin X or nutrient Y, whether or not we have a chronic illness. Therefore navigating our way through this ever-changing catalogue of guidance can be exceptionally difficult, especially coupled with brain fog and fatigue. You may want to visit a dietician, nutritionist or nutritional therapist for help on the best supplements; however, please read the end of this section before spending large sums of money on such consultations. There are without doubt some very good and highly qualified nutrition experts who see private patients, but as with most disciplines, there are also ones who may not have the skills to treat CFS/ME.

As already mentioned, there has not been enough research on CAMs for government healthcare agencies such as NICE to advocate their use. However there are many studies that have investigated the utility of individual supplements for CFS/ME, and you may want to discuss these with your doctor or nutritional therapist.

Magnesium

More than two decades ago a paper was published in the medical journal *The Lancet* that stated that magnesium treatment would benefit people with CFS/ME. This assertion was based on a study that tested levels of magnesium in 20 people with CFS/ME and compared these to people who were matched in terms of age, sex and social class – the latter presumably to account for differences in diet. Because the researchers found that those with CFS/ME had lower levels of magnesium in their blood, a subsequent study gave 15 people magnesium injections for six weeks and 17 people a placebo treatment. The people who had the magnesium therapy said their energy levels had improved, pain had subsided and also that their emotional state seemed better. Magnesium levels returned to normal in all of the individuals receiving the magnesium treatment, but only in one person given a placebo treatment. The reason why at least some people with CFS/ME have lowered magnesium levels is still unclear but we do know that a number of stress hormones can negatively affect tissue magnesium levels. Magnesium supplementation is safe within the recommended daily intake (RDI) amounts. When you look at a supplement container it will often state the RDI, so you can see how much of a particular substance is in a supplement capsule. Unless you have been given expert advice to exceed this amount it is best to stay within this guidance.

Vitamin B12

In 1993 Dr Charles Lapp, a doctor based in North Carolina, provided a rationale for the use of high-dose vitamin B12, also known as cobalamin. This statement was published in the Chronicle of Physicians' Forum for the Chronic Fatigue and Immune Dysfunction Syndrome (CFIDS) Association, which is the USA's main charity for CFS/ME. It was observed that 30 per cent of people with CFS/ME had B12 deficiency when using a highly sensitive test. In another small-scale study of 12 women who met the diagnostic criteria for both CFS/ME and fibromyalgia, levels of vitamin B12 were associated with reported fatigue – that is, those with the highest fatigue symptoms had the lowest levels of vitamin B12. Anecdotally, for instance in online patient forums and support groups, some people who have been given vitamin B12 injections have said that they felt some improvements immediately afterwards but that these gains seemed to wear off and were not noticed again with repeated injections. Hence there is not yet enough evidence to show that vitamin B12 deficiency is a central issue in CFS/ME and one that can be remedied by supplementation. However as with any deficiencies, if you do have tests that show you are deficient in a vitamin or nutrient, it may be beneficial to take supplements.

Essential fatty acids

Essential fatty acids (EFAs), are important for maintaining good physical and mental health, but our bodies cannot produce them on their own – we need to ingest sufficient amounts of EFAs from our diet. The two main types of EFAs are omega-3 and omega-6 fatty acids, both of which are found in foods such as fish, leafy vegetables, seeds – for example pumpkin and sunflower – and walnuts. In 1990 a study used high doses of EFAs as a treatment for CFS/ME. Sixty-three people with CFS/ME were either given eight 500 mg capsules of EFAs every day for three months or placebo capsules. When the participants in this study were assessed in terms of fatigue, pain, concentration and depression after one month of treatment, nearly 75 per cent of those taking the EFAs reported improvements whereas 25 per cent of those who had been given the placebo said their symptoms had reduced. Three months after treatment, 85 per cent of those taking EFAs said their symptoms had diminished, whereas only 17 per cent of the placebo group continued to report improvements – this would be expected as the 'placebo effect' wears off. In addition those with abnormally low levels of EFAs at the start of the study saw their levels return to within normal range following treatment. Indeed low levels of EFAs in people with CFS/ME have been found in a number of studies. It has been suggested that viruses may impair EFA metabolism, leading to immune, endocrine and sympathetic nervous system dysfunctions. If you want to have your EFA levels tested, this can be done via private laboratories. These can be expensive, so please discuss this with your healthcare practitioner, whether this is your GP or a nutrition expert. You will need support in interpreting such test results and most private labs will only analyse patient samples when accompanied by some sort of referral, whether privately gained or from your GP. A further word of caution here: overtesting has its dangers too, not only in terms of the impact on your wallet but also with regard to further disappointments – that is, continually receiving 'normal' results. This is why it is vital that you have a good nutritional therapist who will advise you to be tested just for deficiencies that relate to your own specific symptom profile and support you in digesting the results. Please see the end of this section for tips on how to find a reliable CAM practitioner. If you find that your EFA levels are low then supplementation with fish oils and/or evening primrose oil may be beneficial to your overall health and in combating CFS/ME.

L-carnitine

L-carnitine is a necessary compound in muscle metabolism and mitochondrial energy production. As we discussed in Chapter 4, some researchers and doctors believe that mitochondrial dysfunction may be a core issue in CFS/ME. Some studies have found clinically relevant carnitine deficiency in people with CFS/ME while others have illustrated a relationship between carnitine levels and both CFS/ME symptoms and ability to function. In a study published in 2004, three groups of 30 people given different forms of carnitine were observed over eight weeks. All groups experienced benefits in terms of reduced fatigue and improvements in cognitive symptoms such as attention and concentration. However some people in this study reported side effects of overstimulation and sleeplessness and so withdrew from the research. Dr Sigita Plioplys of the Ann and Robert H. Lurie Children's Hospital of Chicago has suggested that only a third of people with CFS/ME may be 'carnitine responders'. Dr Plioplys has also suggested that in those who do respond, improvements can be dramatic, but regrettably levels of L-carnitine in individuals before treatment can't predict how they will respond. L-carnitine is a common supplement nowadays and can be bought at healthfood stores.

Co-enzyme Q10

Co-enzyme Q10, or CoQ10, is also a substance involved in mitochondrial function as well as acting as an antioxidant. In a study of 20 women with CFS/ME who experienced severe post-exertional fatigue (to such a degree that they needed bedrest following just low intensity exercise), it was found that 80 per cent had a CoQ10 deficiency. This deficiency worsened after the women exercised. Following a three-month treatment of 100 mg CoQ10 a day, the amount of exercise the women could do more than doubled. Even the women in the study who did not see such dramatic improvements did report at least some increased exercise tolerance. Regarding CFS/ME symptoms, after three months of CoQ10 supplementation 90 per cent of those in the study reported reductions in fatigue and other symptoms, while 85 per cent had decreased post-exertional fatigue. Like the other supplements mentioned in this chapter, CoQ10 is a readily available supplement that can be found in healthfood stores and large supermarkets.

Acupuncture

Acupuncture is a therapy that has been used for many thousands of years in countries such as China and Japan, and it is one of the key techniques in traditional Chinese medicine. This type of CAM approach is generally more holistic in nature, meaning that the acupuncturist treating you will be interested not only in your physical symptoms but also possible contributing factors in your illness, such as stress and worry. Therefore on your first visit to an acupuncturist he or she may spend quite some time taking a detailed history. During acupuncture treatment numerous metallic, solid and hair-thin needles are inserted in certain anatomical points on your body, although some acupuncturists use 'electroacupuncture', whereby a small electric current is used to stimulate specific points on the body. The stimulation in acupuncture is believed to influence the flow of the body's vital life force known as 'qi'. Qi is thought to regulate not only our physical health but also our mental, emotional and spiritual well-being. This way of considering health and illness would appear to be fitting for a condition such as CFS/ME that can impact on many areas of a person's life.

Acupuncture has been most studied by researchers for the treatment of pain and has been found to be effective for the treatment of chronic low-back pain and osteoarthritis. In 2008 a group of researchers based in Beijing reviewed the published studies on the use of acupuncture in CFS/ME and concluded that this CAM therapy was effective. But as with most CAM techniques, the quality of the research studies was somewhat poor overall and the authors suggested that more research should be carried out to ensure that acupuncture is indeed a worthwhile treatment option for CFS/ME.

There are relatively few side effects from acupuncture but some people may experience slight soreness, minor bleeding or bruising at the needle sites. A study published in the *British Medical Journal* found that the risk of a serious reaction to acupuncture is less than 1 in 10,000, which would suggest that this type of treatment is safer than many medical procedures. But there can be a risk of infection if the needles are not sterile. Bear in mind that needles should only be used once and are disposable, so if you think the acupuncturist is reusing needles, please terminate treatment. Reusable needles will be wrapped in plastic so it is easy to see if the needles your acupuncturist is using are this type; simply ask to see them at the start of the session. If the needles are not hygienically packaged and disposable, do not continue with treatment. In the UK qualified acupuncturists are registered with the British Acupuncture Council, and you can search for an acupuncturist near you on their website (see the Useful addresses section for details).

Yoga

Yoga is another mind–body approach. It originated in ancient India. This practice is believed to influence the spiritual, mental, emotional and physical aspects of a person. Although historically yoga was associated with religions such as Hinduism and Buddhism, now this gentle moderate form of exercise is often a secular pursuit. In its simplest form yoga is a series of stretching poses carried out with controlled breathing. There are numerous different types of yoga but for people with a condition such as CFS/ME, the most subtle and restorative methods would be best to try. For instance, Ananda yoga uses gentle postures that help with body alignment and can be used as a precursor to meditation. However, you may find yoga classes merely labelled as 'restorative yoga' – these would be more suitable for people with CFS/ME than some of the more demanding methods. Restorative yoga focuses more on relaxation and often uses only a handful of yoga postures in a class. But please note that within all forms of yoga the purpose is to attempt the poses within your own limits rather than pushing yourself to do more than your body is comfortable with. When you join a class, do have a quiet word with the instructor and let her or him know about your health so that you can get proper advice.

Researchers looking at a range of CAM therapies have found that yoga was the most helpful treatment as compared to prescribed medications, non-prescribed supplements and herbs, lifestyle changes, alternative therapies and psychological support for people with unexplained fatigue. However this was for a group of people that included those with unexplained fatigue, not just those with CFS/ME. This means that the people in this study may not have been as severely affected as people who have been diagnosed with CFS/ME – that is, they may have had more energy than a group consisting solely of people with CFS/ME, so the findings should be viewed with caution. There is clearly a need for more research into yoga and CFS/ME, but as yoga has been shown in many studies to be a good relaxation practice, this technique could potentially be used within a pacing programme as a way to relax.

Although yoga is not a regulated practice, there are organizations that can direct you to yoga therapists who have completed a minimal level of training. For example, in the UK the British Council for Yoga Therapy lists a number of member organizations that provide contact information for yoga therapists; in the USA the Yoga Alliance has a search option to find a local practitioner (for both, see Useful addresses).

Meditation and mindfulness

Like yoga, meditation is a form of 'active' relaxation. By practising techniques such as yoga and meditation it is possible to rest the mind and body without sleeping. This is an important aspect of pacing because scheduling-in rest periods is imperative, but simply sitting or lying down may not be restful in itself if your mind continues to race. Mindfulness is a particular type of meditative process that encourages you to be in the moment rather than thinking of the past, worrying about the future or focusing overly on your symptoms. Conversely, trying very hard not to think about symptoms can actually have the opposite effect and make us even more aware of them. To achieve mindful awareness, techniques such as progressive awareness and body scanning can be used. The key to these practices is that your attention should be directed in a completely non-judgemental way. This may seem incredibly unnatural at first as we innately try to evaluate incoming information – it is simply part of being human. However, when attempting meditation and mindfulness, the trick is to have awareness of a sensation without trying to dissect it. Like any skill, perfecting meditation and mindfulness is a progressive endeavour and will take some dedication. If you can allocate time to meditate on a daily basis it can become an integral part of your life and certainly won't seem like a task; rather, the time you spend in mindful awareness should be peaceful, enjoyable and something to look forward to.

In addition to acting as a form of relaxation, mindfulness and meditation may help to deal with the dysfunction in the hypothalamic–pituitary–adrenal (HPA) axis that has been observed in people with CFS/ME (as outlined in Chapter 4). Research investigating improvements following taught sessions of mindfulness in groups of people – not only with CFS/ME but also fibromyalgia and multiple chemical sensitivity – have found that this approach can reduce anxiety, depression and also pain. Furthermore in a study of breast and prostate cancer patients, changes in some physiological measures associated with the HPA axis were found after eight weeks of a programme that combined mindfulness, meditation and yoga.

There are countless websites that give examples of meditation and mindfulness exercises. There are also numerous CDs and books on the topic that can be bought at any bookshop with a health and well-being section (or sometimes they are placed in the self-help section) or online. Free smartphone and tablet apps are also available, although often these have a paid option to access further exercises. However, you may want to join a class as it can be helpful to have the opportunity to ask questions and learn from someone who can help to tailor the exercises to you and the stage of your illness. For example, if you are very limited in energy you may want to start with short, perhaps only two-minute sessions that can be increased over time when your health improves.

Hypnotherapy

Hypnotherapy is another technique that may help to break free from the chronic stress some people with CFS/ME experience, either before they became ill or as a result of it. The hypnotherapist will use 'hypnotic induction' to help you reach a hypnotic state. Techniques used are similar to those in meditation and mindfulness in the sense that they are progressive. For instance, in guided imagery the hypnotherapist leads you on a journey in your mind to a peaceful and safe place, such as a clearing in a forest or a secret garden. Once you have reached a hypnotic state you will be in a state of not only deep relaxation but also heightened awareness. Here you will be focusing exclusively on the hypnotherapist's voice and it is at this point that the therapist can suggest ideas and concepts that may be able to break the stress loop that some people with CFS/ME have. Considering that CFS/ME can be such a debilitating illness that impacts on all areas of life, feeling generalized anxiety is not an atypical consequence. As with all of the CAM treatments outlined in this chapter, hypnotherapy does not constitute a cure for CFS/ME but it might help deal with stress, which can in turn help our immune systems to function at their best. Here Hayley describes her experience of hypnotherapy:

> I had a hypnotherapy session where the aim was to strengthen my immune system. I was continually having colds, every couple of weeks, and had flu-like symptoms most of the time. Under hypnosis I was asked to visualize building up a brick wall that was symbolizing my immune system. Coincidence or not, but after this I no longer had many colds. I still had flu-like symptoms, including fluctuating temperature and sore throat, but I no longer had full-blown snotty colds. Sadly this had no effect on my ME, and my fatigue kept getting worse. (Hayley)

At present the research for the utility of hypnotherapy in CFS/ME is very thin on the ground. However some studies looking at related conditions such as fibromyalgia and irritable bowel syndrome indicate that this technique can relieve illness-related symptoms as well as fatigue, pain and sleep difficulties. Clearly, though, there is a need for specific studies with people who have CFS/ME.

In the UK, you can locate a qualified hypnotherapist via the Hypnotherapy Association UK, the National Hypnotherapy Society and the General Hypnotherapy Register websites (see Useful addresses). It is also worth bearing in mind that an increasing number of health-care professionals are trained in hypnotherapy and may be able to offer you this treatment. For instance, the American Society of Clinical Hypnosis has members who are psychologists, psychiatrists, clinical social workers, marriage and family therapists, mental health counsellors, medical doctors, masters-level nurses, dentists and chiropractors. So you could discuss hypnotherapy with your GP or specialist, who may be able to refer you to a professional who offers hypnotherapy.

General advice on finding a CAM practitioner

Although there are various registers and organizations that represent CAM practitioners, this area is not as highly regulated as traditional medicine, hence a certain degree of care should be taken when choosing a therapist. In the UK the Complementary and Natural Healthcare Council (CNHC) is a voluntary organization that regulates CAM practitioners. The CNHC is backed by the UK government and is approved by the Professional Standards Authority for Health and Social Care. However, practitioners are not legally obliged to be part of this regulatory body – it is voluntary, so there are a large number of therapists not registered with the CNHC for a range of reasons (for example, they may not have the necessary training required for registration or they may simply not wish to be part of such an organization). Nevertheless it is a good idea to ask a therapist if she or he is part of a regulatory body. Other tips when selecting a CAM practitioner include:

- Ask for details of the practitioner's qualifications. Some seemingly impressive qualifications can be based on quite an insignificant amount of training, for instance a weekend-long course. Use a web search engine to track down the qualifications or letters after therapists' names to make sure they have completed rigorous study.
- A personal recommendation can be a strong suggestion that the practitioner is worthy of your business – do remember that health-care is a business – but don't rely on testimonials from a website. The Advertising Standards Authority in the UK has quite strict guidelines on the evidence needed for practitioners to make health claims. Testimonials are not seen to be valid forms of proof for the benefits of therapies in defined conditions such as CFS/ME. Therefore ask practitioners what evidence there is to support their practice.

- If anyone tells you that he or she has a '100-per-cent success rate' in treating people with CFS/ME, run a mile! Likewise, if a practitioner states that a certain technique is a 'cure' for CFS/ME, he or she is not fit to treat you as there is no known cure for this condition.
- If a therapist is pushy or tries to give you a hard sell, do not hand over any money. Anyone who is good at treating people will not need to do this. All forms of healthcare are expensive so don't be persuaded into paying large sums of money if you don't feel exceptionally confident about the practitioner's background and abilities.

Chloe neatly sums up these tips for finding a CAM therapist:

> Although I have used conventional medicine while having ME, I prefer to treat the root cause of symptoms. So I have used homeopathy, emotional freedom technique, spiritual healing, acupuncture, neurolinguistic programming and more. However, there are dangers with such practitioners. Some, besides charging an enormous amount of money, have very little experience. I have seen them out of their depth. Always ask about a person's training and maybe the amount of clients the practitioner has or any questions you want to ask before committing yourself to a course of treatment. Get a personal recommendation if you can and at least find out about the therapist's qualifications. Some people do exceedingly short courses before declaring themselves Masters. On the other hand, you might find a beginner and be happy with the cost. (Chloe)

Of course, even if you have done your research on the therapist this does not mean the treatment will definitely work for you. Because CFS/ME is such a variable condition, some things can help some symptoms for some people and not for others. This can be disheartening and also exhausting. Therefore only try one technique at a time. This is also important because if you are attempting 101 treatments at the same time it will be impossible to know which one has produced the benefits.

Summary and conclusion

In this chapter we have outlined some of the CAM treatments most commonly reported by people with CFS/ME. As mentioned at the beginning of this chapter, this list is not exhaustive and new techniques are continually being created and offered for those with fatiguing conditions such as CFS/ME. There is a need for more research to evaluate not only the effectiveness of these and other techniques but also the mechanisms by which they work, if indeed they do. Hence the inclusion of the approaches in this chapter does not amount to an endorsement – the information included here is simply for you to use as a springboard if you so wish. In the next chapter we will look at a number of everyday techniques that you can use to improve your health in general.

9

Additional things you can do to help your condition

In addition to seeing your doctor and trying medicines to help with particular symptoms, and perhaps engaging in a programme of activity management and/or investigating alternative therapies and supplements, there are various techniques you can use yourself, at home. In this chapter we will describe a number of strategies, some of which are common sense and some you may not have heard of before you had CFS/ME.

Regular routines

When you are in the most severe stages of CFS/ME, perhaps following an infection or an acutely stressful event such as looking after a sick relative, it may not be possible to introduce regular routines. But if you are further along in your illness, perhaps having improved after a programme of pacing, it is beneficial to try to develop routines. CFS/ME can make you feel out of control and the symptoms can be unpredictable, certainly when people are first ill and don't know much about the illness. By setting daily routines you can take back a sense of control and also keep symptoms at bay. While this is common sense, of course it can be difficult to do with a chronic illness. If you can, try to:

- Set a sleep routine by going to bed and waking up at the same time each day. Unless you are in the initial phase of the illness, try not to sleep in the day but instead set rest periods – see below for more on ways to rest without sleeping – as daily naps can disturb night-time sleep. This, unfortunately, can lead to a vicious circle of not getting enough good-quality sleep at night, which leads to feeling exhausted in the day – so much so that you need a nap but then because you have slept in the day you can't get to sleep at night. If your sleep cycle is very badly disturbed, consider a technique called 'sleep restriction', discussed below, which can help to reset your sleep–wake cycle.

- Schedule meals at regular time-periods. Some people with CFS/ ME have symptoms similar to hypoglycaemia – that is, low blood sugar. These symptoms include trembling, clammy skin, heart palpitations (pounding or fast heartbeats), sweating, hunger and irritability, which are relieved when blood sugar levels are normalized. Blood sugar levels can be regulated not only by when but also by what you eat – try to eat foods high in protein such as meat, eggs, tofu, cheese, nuts and seeds. Also, slow-release carbohydrates such as non-starchy vegetables (spinach, kale, tomatoes, broccoli, cauliflower, cucumber, onions and asparagus), sweet potatoes, and quinoa can help maintain even blood sugar levels. Avoiding high-sugar, processed foods such as cakes, cookies, biscuits and fizzy drinks can also help because consuming these can lead to sugar spikes, which are followed by blood sugar crashes. But as with all the advice in this book, make sure you have treats – the stress of keeping too strictly to healthy eating can be counterproductive and, well, we all need a cake occasionally! Finally, add in regular snacks such as a handful of nuts or hummus to maintain blood sugar levels and prevent that ravenous feeling that may lead to a raiding of the biscuit tin.
- If you are taking medication it can be helpful to set reminders on your phone or a repeating alarm. Even for someone without brain fog this can help. It can also be useful to use a pill box with separate compartments for each day because tasks that we do every day can often merge together in our minds. If we do the same thing at the same time every day it can be difficult to know if we have taken tablets today or if the memory trace is a combined memory from numerous days; this is why the contraceptive pill has days written on the pack as it is all too easy for medication use to feel like *Groundhog Day*.

But a routine shouldn't just be about the everyday necessities. When you are recovering, include activities you enjoy in your daily plan. This can be even more important than the above advice since having something to look forward to every day, regardless of CFS/ME, is vital for our well-being. Which activity you choose may be related to your current energy levels, remembering of course that even using a computer can be tiring – for some more than taking a walk. Art-making can be therapeutic in itself and can take countless forms. Some people with CFS/ME make cards that are then sold by charities to raise funds. Genealogy can also be a pleasurable pastime and there are now quite a few websites that help with tracking your family tree. Cooking or baking has also been said to facilitate recovery in people who have the physical energy to do this:

> After I was no longer bedbound with ME, I found that cooking really helped me. I think it was because I had to concentrate on something but there was no pressure like with schoolwork. I had a high stool in the kitchen, which I used to make sure it wasn't too much for me, and I chose relatively easy recipes at the start. I love making things for people so I would bake things like brownies and biscuits for when my friends would come over. By then there were only a few friends who came to see me but this was all right as they were the ones who counted. I felt I could sort of pay them back for the effort they made to come and see me with the biscuits, so it felt like cooking was something I could do for other people. So I think it had a double purpose for me, not just to take my mind off the CFS/ME but it also helped to have something else to talk about with my friends as I wasn't going to school at the time. And they seemed pretty happy to eat the brownies! (Amy)

Sleep restriction

As noted in Chapter 5, researchers have found that a high proportion of people with CFS/ME have sleep disorders. If this is the case then the primary sleep disorder should be diagnosed and treated. However, a great many people with CFS/ME have trouble sleeping even if they do not have a diagnosable sleep disorder. Conversely, when you are first ill you may feel the need to sleep throughout the day. This is called hypersomnia, as opposed to insomnia, which is when you cannot fall asleep or stay asleep – the latter is a more recognizable term as it is more prevalent in the general population than hypersomnia. While it is important to support the body when it is fighting an infection or dealing with trauma, after the first acute period of illness, when hyper-somnia is unpreventable (that is, the need to sleep is overwhelming, as during a flu infection), it is best to try to avoid daytime naps. As noted in the pacing session, incorporating rest and relaxation times is imperative when sustaining a baseline and increasing activities, but actual sleep can disturb your sleep–wake cycle.

Before outlining general tips for sleep, here is a technique known as 'sleep restriction' that you may want to use if your sleep patterns are very erratic. We all have an internal body clock that helps us to know when to sleep and when to rise. As we have noted a couple of times in passing, the 24-hour sleep–wake cycle is known as the circadian rhythm. Although this cycle is mostly controlled by internal processes and hormones, external factors such as light and temperature can also play a part in when we wake up and sleep.

Sleep restriction can be useful as a way of resetting the circadian rhythm or body clock if it has become out of kilter. But please note that this is a temporary measure to regain a good sleep pattern and should not be used indefinitely. Before you start restricting your amount of sleep, you need to calculate your current sleep efficiency. This can be done by dividing the time you are asleep by the time you spend in bed and multiplying this by 100 – that is, time asleep ÷ time-in-bed × 100. This will result in a percentage. Most healthy people get around 90 per cent sleep efficiency but for people with exceptionally disrupted sleep efficiency can be as low as 5 per cent. An example of the sleep effi-ciency calculation is that is if you are in bed for eight hours but only sleep six hours, your sleep efficiency is 75 per cent – that is, 6 ÷ 8 × 100 = 75 per cent. Sleep efficiency should only be calculated for time-in-bed at night, not for any time-in-bed during the day. Therefore if you have very severe CFS/ME and are bedbound, this calculation will not apply to you – in general, sleep restriction is not recommended for people with severe CFS/ME, but if you do have severe CFS/ME and want to try this technique, discuss it with your doctor.

To calculate your average sleep time, monitor yourself for two weeks. You can do this simply by noting down the amount of time you've spent in bed and the amount of time you think you've actually slept, or you can download a sleep app on a smartphone if you have one. There are free sleep apps and also ones that need to be purchased.

Also, before starting your sleep restriction, ensure a regular rising time – for every day of every week, set your clock to wake you at a time you think is in tune with your body. This differs for different people. You may have heard the expressions 'morning lark' and 'night owl': research shows that some people are indeed naturally early risers while others' body clocks are set later in the day. Therefore don't try to force your-self into a pattern you've never had, even before you became ill with CFS/ME. This may be 8 a.m. for you or 10 a.m.; the important thing is that before you commence sleep restriction, your body gets accustomed again to waking up at the same time every day, even at the weekends.

To start your sleep restriction you need to limit the time you spend in bed to the number of hours you actually sleep. Hence if you spend eight hours in bed but you have found that you only actually sleep for five hours on average, you start the sleep restriction programme by being in bed for five hours only. This needs to be set with regard to your natural wake time, so if you have been waking up at 8 a.m. with your alarm clock, you need to go to bed at 3 a.m. This may appear to be completely counterintuitive if you're exhausted, but sleep restriction is a way to regain a more normal sleep–wake cycle. This initial step in sleep restriction is no doubt difficult, and you will need to be disciplined to carry out the programme, which can feel dreadful at first. It might be easier to set a wake time of 6 a.m. so that you only have to stay up until 1 a.m. – you need to decide what is best for you and what you can handle.

Reducing time-in-bed works because it increases prior wakefulness, and by the time you get to 1 a.m. or even 3 a.m. and are still awake, you are really tired – although we know we are tired a lot of the time anyway. Next, when you wake up in the morning you calculate your sleep efficiency again – time asleep ÷ time-in-bed × 100. All being well your sleep efficiency will have risen somewhat. If so, for a week stick to just five hours in bed, but if you find you are in bed for five hours but only sleep for say four hours, you will need to reduce the time-in-bed to four hours. But if you sleep for five hours after monitoring for a week, then you can allow yourself an extra 15 minutes (or 30 minutes – this is flexible) in bed, thus going to bed at 12.45 a.m. if previously you were going to bed at 1 a.m.

Then, if you sleep for five hours and 15 minutes for the next couple of weeks – while still monitoring your sleep efficiency – you can increase your time-in-bed further. You need to aim for the sleep efficiency that you think is reasonable. Aiming for 90 per cent when you have CFS/ME, which is an illness with known sleep problems, may be unrealistic. You may also not have been a very good sleeper before you had CFS/ME, so trying to obtain very high sleep efficiency may actually be damaging if it is an out-of-reach goal. A better goal may be aiming for between 75 and 85 per cent sleep efficiency. The programme should be carried out slowly and gently over six weeks, and once you have reached a good proportion of sleep to time-in-bed, keep to this pattern. With any luck your daytime wakefulness will be improved and possibly some other CFS/ME symptoms will diminish.

General advice on sleep

Even if you don't have substantially disrupted sleep, good 'sleep hygiene' practice is something that you can do to support your immune system in general because lack of sleep can dampen the immune response. Here are a few general tips that everyone can follow, not just people with CFS/ME:

- Your evening meal may affect your ability to sleep. A heavy meal just before bed can disturb sleep as your body digests the food, so if your large meal of the day is an evening meal, try to have this in the early part of the evening. However, going to bed hungry is also disruptive, so if you're hungry, a light snack before bed is better than not eating. In general, high-protein foods are best at lunchtime (such as meat, fish, eggs) and carbohydrate-rich foods (pasta, bread, potatoes and so on) are good in the evening. Eating carbohydrates leads to the release of the neurotransmitter serotonin – in Chapter 6 we saw how some antidepressants work by impeding the reabsorption of serotonin. The same mechanism may be at play here when we eat carbohydrate-laden foods.
- In addition to avoiding large meals just before bed it is also a good idea to leave out that cup of coffee after your last meal of the day. Caffeine, of course, is a stimulant and so keeps us awake. Coffee, tea, cola and other fizzy drinks contain high levels of caffeine, as does chocolate. But you can buy some very good caffeine-free alternatives these days, so you don't have to go without your favourite beverages. Coffee lovers will often have their 'good' cup of caffeinated coffee in the morning, then stick to decaffeinated versions later in the day. Even though it may seem counterintuitive, alcohol can prevent us from having a good night's sleep. Although a nightcap may initially make us feel drowsy, the alcohol will disrupt later stages of sleep because our bodies have to metabolize it. This can result in waking up in the middle of the night.
- This may sound like an old wives' tale, but hot baths just before bed do help some people fall asleep. This may be because after a bath our bodies are hot and then gradually cool down, rather than being cold and requiring time and energy to increase their temperature. Some people find showers quite invigorating, so if you have a tub, try soaking in the bath rather than taking a hot shower.
- It is important to create a bedroom that is conducive for sleep. Gentle lighting can help with this, as can an optimum temperature. How hot or cool we like our bedrooms is a personal choice, but in general a freezing cold or boiling hot environment does not help us to sleep. If you live somewhere quiet, consider leaving a window open so that there is enough fresh air and oxygen

circulating the room – a stuffy room can impede a good night's sleep.

- If outside noise is an issue for you, noise machines can help to block out any external sounds. There is a wide range of these available now, with various different settings. Some have natural sounds like ocean waves crashing, rainfall, a beating heart and birdsong. Others use 'white noise' that sounds a bit like static on a television. While it may seem odd to add more noise to your environment if noise itself is keeping you awake, noise machines can be beneficial because they emit constant and soothing sound rather than abrupt noise. A fan can also act as a noise machine, and has the added advantage of circulating air in the bedroom.

- If noise machines don't suit you, you may want to invest in some good-quality earplugs. Bespoke earplugs can be purchased from larger chemists. These should last many years but they are expensive. You will need to make an appointment and have moulds taken of your ears – these will then be sent off so that the plugs can be made to fit your ears perfectly. The process can take a few weeks, however, so you may want to buy some inexpensive earplugs in the meantime. Indeed it may be a good idea to start off with these cheaper versions to see if they suit you before investing in bespoke ones. Inexpensive earplugs are usually made from foam or silicone, so if you have an allergy to silicone take a careful look at the packaging.

- When settling down for the night, try to steer clear of highly stimulating television programmes, music and video games. In fact it's best to ban 'screens' from the bedroom – this includes computers and smartphones. If our brains are constantly engaged and alert it can be hard to switch off. However, if you are bedbound with CFS/ME and your contact with the outside world is via the internet, then it may be difficult to delineate the bedroom for sleeping only. If this is the case, do still attempt to limit screen-time in terms of your pacing schedule.

- Earlier we discussed the sleep–wake cycle or circadian rhythm. Natural light is vital for this cycle but this can be hard to get enough of if you're limited to indoor activities. If you can, try simply to sit outside for a period of time, or if you are well enough, a brief walk can be beneficial. This will also help you to acquire vitamin D, which people can be deficient in if they are not exposed to enough natural light. There are numerous types of 'light boxes' on sale currently, which may also help maintain your circadian rhythm, but outdoor light is best where possible.

- Light boxes also exist that act as alarm clocks. They operate by gradually increasing the light they emit, mirroring a sunrise. Some people with CFS/ME find this a much more calming way to wake up. At night they work in the opposite direction, starting off relatively bright and slowly dimming. This may be another gadget you'd like to try.
- Depending on your level of activity, gentle exercise like yoga can help improve sleep quality. This may also be due to the meditative state and deep relaxation that yoga can produce.

You may want to try some, or all, of the above techniques to help you sleep well. However, a note of caution: gadgets such as noise machines and light boxes/alarm clocks, as well as the bespoke earplugs, can mount up in terms of cost, so you may want to try one at a time. Check the return policy for gadgets – there may be a free trial period. In the next section, other simple techniques you can use to help you relax will be described, which can also help with sleep quality.

Dealing with worry and rumination

In Chapter 6 we briefly described a treatment for CFS/ME called cognitive behavioural therapy (CBT). One aim of CBT is to help break any repetitive and negative thought patterns, sometimes referred to as 'rumination'. Constant worry and rumination can be exhausting in itself and so it can certainly help your day-to-day life if repetitive negative thought patterns are broken. But this by no means implies that breaking thought patterns is a cure for CFS/ME; rather, using strategies to diminish worry and rumination can improve the quality of life not only for people with illnesses such as CFS/ME but for everyone.

One of the most common things to ruminate about when having CFS/ME is whether you will recover. Thoughts like 'I will never get better' and 'I no longer have control over my body and my life' can roam around in your head over and over again. These kinds of thoughts are perfectly normal and unsurprising in an illness such as CFS/ME, which can seem unpredictable and never-ending. They're particularly common if you've experienced a setback in your pacing programme – that is, your symptoms have worsened when trying to increase activity. Here it is important to take a step back and know this is simply a temporary setback on the path to recovery. Increasing the amount you can comfortably do is a process that may feel at times 'two steps forward, one step back'. Focus on the positives – if you're just starting with a pacing programme then you've already come far because you now know your baseline level of activity. This in itself is an achievement – you're taking control over your illness and your life. Before you knew your baseline you would not have known how much activity was reasonable in your current condition, which is why your symptoms may have spiked at times. By looking at your activity diary objectively it is possible to begin to see patterns in your symptom spikes, sometimes called crashes. These will most probably have been caused by doing more than your energy level allows. So if you have a setback and begin to ruminate about whether you will ever recover, tell yourself that you are actively taking back control of your body and your life. Also, if you are further along in your pacing programme and have had setbacks before, remember that you have recovered from previous crashes and focus on the time before your symptoms worsened – you would have only increased your activity if you felt able.

Another repetitive thought you may have concerns self-blame. CFS/ ME is a condition in which the exact cause is still unknown. This is probably because there are many causes, which differ between people – as discussed in Chapters 3 and 4, explanatory models of CFS/ME include a number of different factors, not just one. However, having CFS/ME is not your fault. You did not seek out this illness and you are not to blame for having it. If you are reading this book, you are actively trying to improve your situation. If others make you feel that you are to blame for becoming ill, halt these negative thoughts by accepting that CFS/ME can be hard for other people to understand. You are no more to blame for having CFS/ME than someone with cancer is to blame for that.

Similarly, repeatedly questioning what single thing caused your illness can also be a ruminative thought. Replaying the past in our minds is rarely helpful. We cannot change the past and even if we could there is not a definite trigger for everyone with CFS/ME. Frankly, even if your illness was triggered by an infection there would have been very little you could have done to prevent contracting it. This is not to say you shouldn't take good care of yourself in the future and draw something constructive from having a condition such as CFS/ME, though of course this may only be possible after you have experienced at least a degree of recovery. For instance, if you have always put others before yourself, this may be an opportunity to recognize that you need to prioritize yourself, at least some of the time. You may have been particularly engrossed in your career and now feel that other areas of life are also valuable, such as family and friends. There may have been a pastime you always wanted to pursue but never felt you had the time. You may take this period as an opportunity to change the course of your life in subtle ways. If you are in the most severe phase of your illness this may be impossible to contemplate, but directing your attention to things in which you find pleasure and satisfaction can shed new light on your circumstances:

> It is more than 30 years since I started to draw tiny cartoons with quotations beneath them. It was those tiny pictures and positive thoughts that took me forward. Since then I use my creativity to distract myself in many ways, be it art, poetry, children's stories or research on this or that for a long-term project I may have started. Most importantly I have to remember to be kind to myself and that I have choices. Creativity can lead me to new heights I had never expected – let my choices take me forward today. (Mary)

Finally, when we can't do what we would like to do it can be easy to be very critical of ourselves. We all do the best we can in the situation we're in. If you find that you're berating yourself for not being good enough, not being able to do everything you did before you had CFS/ME and not being a good mother/father/son/daughter/worker any more, tell yourself that it is all right not to be perfect in all these things. It is crucial that you take any unnecessary pressure off yourself while you are recovering. Having an illness such as CFS/ME can often lead us to reappraise our beliefs and values. Before you had CFS/ME, doing things 'just so' may have seemed vital, but is it now? Very few situations are critical and, in truth, no one else may notice if you've let the housework pile up or haven't responded to an email straight away – other people are too worried about themselves and their lives. Show yourself the compassion you undoubtedly extend to others.

> When I try too hard to please other people I forget to pace myself. Pacing myself means taking care of me and what is important in my own life, even though I want to help others in theirs. I have to remind myself that pacing is about progress, not perfection. I will take care of me today. (Mary)

Social support

Social support refers to the help and assistance received from others; this can take many forms and is not necessarily easy to put into words. Social support could be overt support such as financial assistance or help with tasks such as gardening and shopping. It can simply be advice and guidance or something more emotionally supportive such as listening or counselling – or even just a sense of belonging. There are formal and informal types of social support: the former are usually provided by a professional (such as a social worker, paid carer or advocate), the latter often by friends, family and co-workers. There is a wealth of research that shows how important social support is for maintaining well-being. Its lack can impact not only on psychological but also physical health. Furthermore research by Professors Ronald Glaser and Janice Kiecolt-Glaser, who were introduced in Chapter 4, has shown that low levels of social support can impact negatively on immune-system functioning. Therefore gaining, and maintaining, support networks is definitely something to consider, whether you have CFS/ME or not.

Of course, this can be much easier said than done. As there is not a biomedical test for CFS/ME, such as a blood test, some people may not believe that you have a 'real' illness. As we saw in Chapter 1, CFS/ME has had an extraordinarily bumpy past and also, because people with the condition often look well, it can be difficult for others to understand. In general, if someone has a strong belief that CFS/ME is 'all in the mind' it probably isn't worth using your limited energy to change his or her mind. This can be termed a negative social support and is not conducive to recovery. Similarly, if a friend or loved one tells you to 'Pull yourself together' or 'If I were you, I'd get myself up and get on with life', you may wish to disengage and focus on your recovery. However, there will be people who do understand the illness; they may not comprehend it absolutely but they will appreciate that you are unwell and in need of support.

With those people who are able to support you it is essential to be honest and say what you need. Most of us find it awfully hard to ask for help, but you should see it as a core part of your recovery programme rather than that you're weak/not good enough/a failure. If you have children the most fundamental assistance may be having a friend help with the school run. If you live alone you may benefit from a volunteer service that can help with jobs around the house. But perhaps most of all, the companionship and understanding of others with CFS/ME can be valuable. This is where local support groups help.

While the thought of joining a group where the only thing you have in common is an illness may not seem attractive, meeting people who are or have gone through the same experiences as you can be quite enlightening. Also, treatment approaches and therapies are often discussed in support-group meetings. There are far more treatments and therapies than the space in this book allows us to consider, so support groups can provide routes to new and useful information. If you are not well enough to attend face-to-face meetings, most groups have paper newsletters and/or online forums. If you can't locate your nearest group via an online search, contact your national CFS/ME organization, which should have lists of local groups.

National charities also offer formal advice and advocacy. In the UK the two largest CFS/ME organizations, the ME Association and Action for ME (AfME), offer a range of support services. The ME Association provides over 30 information booklets and leaflets relating to treatment, ranging from explanation of blood-test results to managing emotions. AfME also publishes numerous information sheets, although this organization concentrates more on the topics of lifestyle management and cognitive-behavioural approaches, such as 'controlling symptoms'.

CFS/ME, like many other invisible illnesses, can be incredibly isolating, but you are not alone. If your pre-illness support networks are no longer there, reach out – there are people who can support you, whether in a practical, informational or emotional sense.

Summary and conclusion

In this chapter we have discussed some additional strategies you can incorporate in your daily life that will not only help you in your recovery but also enable you to remain well when the CFS/ME symptoms subside. For everyone, not just those with illnesses such as CFS/ME, regular routines, good sleep quality, dealing with worry and rumination and accessing positive social support are good ways to stay healthy in a world that is often full of constant stimulation and stresses.

10

The future of CFS/ME

In Chapter 1 we took a very brief journey through the history of CFS/ME, from the documentation of a disorder known as neurasthenia in the mid-1800s to the present-day conception of chronic fatigue syndrome. Our understanding of the condition has undoubtedly been influenced by cultural, political and societal beliefs and values, which often impact on such important decisions as the allocation of funding for research and healthcare. This chapter will outline recent developments in terms of research and the changing perception of CFS/ME, which will, we hope, show that progress has been made in the past two decades.

The UK CFS/ME Research Collaborative

In April 2013 the UK CFS/ME Research Collaborative was launched in London. The purpose of this collaborative was to bring together researchers, charities and funders in an effort to increase awareness of CFS/ME in the research and scientific community and also to persuade funders of the value of supporting research into this condition. From 2008 to 2011 an expert group from the Medical Research Council (one of the biggest research funding bodies in the UK), and led by Professor Stephen Holgate, had been looking at ways to increase the amount of research into CFS/ME. The idea for a collaborative stemmed from the achievements of the UK Respiratory Research Collaborative, which proved to be very successful in encouraging new researchers to investigate this area and funders to allocate funds for this work. The London launch was very well attended and included presentations from current researchers and healthcare professionals in the area. In addition to raising awareness, the objectives of the collaborative included:

- To help facilitate a range of high-quality research in both adults and children. The types of research identified at the launch comprised basic science studies looking at the underlying mechanisms of the disorder (for example, immune function), research to clarify the types and numbers of people affected by CFS/ME (that is, epidemiological studies), research looking at what kinds of health services people with CFS/ME use and studies evaluating treatment and prevention programmes for the condition.

- To encourage different types of researchers and doctors to work together in multidisciplinary teams.
- To encourage professional and industrial organizations to link up with researchers and doctors in the CFS/ME field.
- To help build an infrastructure for research – for example, technology, databases of people with CFS/ME and resources such as blood and tissue banks for researchers to access.
- To aid the creation of attractive career paths for professionals who would like to be involved with CFS/ME research and healthcare.
- To engender an environment in which more research can be carried out in the National Health Service.
- To highlight the achievements of the CFS/ME research community.
- To liaise with international groups so that information can be shared and further collaborations created.

Membership of this collaborative was open to all UK-based doctors, all other healthcare professionals, researchers and charities involved in CFS/ME research. It is too early to assess its impact, but communication between researchers, doctors, funders and industrial partners can only be a good thing.

Biobanks

One of the goals set out by the UK CFS/ME Research Collaborative is already being pursued. In 2008 the ME Association and Action for ME co-funded a feasibility study into a tissue bank for CFS/ME. The study consisted of interviews with people with CFS/ME, researchers, doctors and professionals with knowledge of the workings of biobanks. It was found that overall there was support for such a resource, and so in March 2011 further funds were given to the research team based at the London School of Hygiene and Tropical Medicine to construct detailed plans for the implementation of the biobank. By August 2011, ME Research UK and a private donor agreed to support the biobank, and the actual repository was initiated.

The physical biobank is currently housed at the Royal Free Hospital, which is part of University College London. The facility holds blood samples from carefully defined people with CFS/ME. This means that only those who meet the criteria for the condition are permitted to donate blood samples. This is important so that any researchers who use the samples can be certain they are studying people with CFS/ME rather than any other disorder. The research team from the London School of Hygiene and Tropical Medicine will analyse the data collected in respect of the characteristics of the people who gave samples – age, biological sex, symptom severity, length of illness and so on – to give the research community an accurate picture of the group of donors. Following on from this the team will analyse some of the blood samples, and the biobank will be open to other researchers from external institutions to access the biological material. The funding of one million pounds for the London School of Hygiene and Tropical Medicine's team to analyse the samples was secured from the USA's National Institute of Health (its leading medical research agency), which illustrates the confidence that large funders have in a resource such as this. This is a major step forward for research into CFS/ME and highlights the flurry of research activity of recent years.

Stratified medicine

An exciting and growing area in many illnesses – not just CFS/ME – is stratified medicine. Stratified medicine means the tailoring of treatments to individuals. As we discovered in Chapters 6 and 8, certain treatments seem to work for some people with CFS/ME but not for others. It's still unclear why this should be the case, therefore more knowledge is needed about the underlying mechanisms of CFS/ME in different people. It is likely that the overall population of people with CFS/ME can be divided into sub-groups. Numerous researchers have already tried to cluster people into smaller groups on the basis of their symptoms but this has not been as useful as we would have liked. People with CFS/ME tend to fall into severity groups rather than groups with predominately cognitive, sleep or pain problems, as might be expected. Thus it will be more useful to see if those with CFS/ME differ from one another in terms of their immune systems, mitochondria function or abnormalities of the autonomic nervous system, for example. At present there are researchers trying to unpick these issues.

This approach to medicine, both in terms of research and healthcare, is a seemingly good fit with an illness such as CFS/ME. To date we have found neither a single cause of the illness nor a treatment that is effective for everyone. Hence the search for a one-size-fits-all approach to treatment has not worked and more creative and sophisticated endeavours are called for. In addition to this there has been a shift in the way knowledge about conditions is shared and communicated. Previously healthcare professionals would have learnt about illnesses in a traditional way through higher education, and this information would have been passed on to patients. An individual would have experienced symptoms, consulted a GP, who would then have diagnosed a condition and treated it. These days it is often the case that patients themselves will do a great deal of research before visiting their doctors, and in some cases may know more about their illness than their GP. This is a huge swing of power in terms of the doctor–patient relationship, which of course has both drawbacks and benefits. Added to this there is a move within the National Health Service for patients to have greater choice via the Any Qualified Provider (AQP) scheme. This means patients will have input not only into the kind of treatment they receive but also into who will provide it. As this initiative is in its early stages, we do not know what the impact of greater choice and flexibility will be in terms of treatment benefits and usage. However, there is scope for non-traditional therapists to gain contracts under AQP, which may result in some previously private – and expensive – therapies being offered within the UK public healthcare system.

The development of new treatments

In addition to unravelling the underlying mechanisms of CFS/ME and the defining sub-groups among those with CFS/ME, new treatments are being developed and discovered. It should be reiterated that these therapies are not to be seen as one-size-fits-all, rather they may work for some people – the research is still at a very early stage and we do not yet know who will benefit. One drug treatment that has received a great deal of attention in recent years is rituximab. In 2011, researchers in the Department of Oncology and Medical Physics at the Haukeland University Hospital in Norway observed that a patient who had CFS/ME appeared to recover to a great extent following chemotherapy. The reason why this female patient was given chemotherapy was because she had later developed Hodgkin's disease, a type of cancer that originates from the white blood cells. At about four weeks from the start of the chemotherapy the patient was able to go for long walks, which she had not been able to do for ten years, her pain improved and so did her cognitive symptoms. These improvements lasted for around five months before all the CFS/ME symptoms gradually started to return.

The Norwegian researchers were so impressed by this observation that they gave two more patients the rituximab treatment. These additional patients also showed improvements, which again wore off after a few months. A second and third course of the drug was administered and demonstrated the same beneficial effects as the first course. Because of these promising findings the researchers carried out a further study of 30 people with CFS/ME, 15 of whom were given rituximab and the remaining 15 placebo treatment. Of those in the rituximab group, 67 per cent showed moderate to major improvements in fatigue while only 13 per cent of the placebo group stated that their fatigue had diminished. Further clinical studies are now being carried out in Norway and funds are being raised to replicate these studies in the UK. Rituximab may work for some people with CFS/ME who have subtle autoimmune abnormalities. This is because the drug works by removing some B cells that produce antibodies that can attack the body's own tissues. However, because this was a chance finding, there is not enough research to say for certain that some people with CFS/ME have an autoimmune condition. Anecdotal reports have suggested that some people with CFS/ME experience more side effects from this treatment than have been reported in the research studies. Hence further work is certainly needed in this area.

Greater understanding of mind–body interactions and treatments

One final exciting development in the research world that may be relevant for those with CFS/ME are the findings related to approaches such as mindfulness. A study published in the scientific journal *Psychoneuroendocrinology* found that intensive mindfulness practice actually caused changes in genes associated with inflammation and immune function. People who were experienced in mindfulness practice were compared to untrained people engaging in quiet but non-meditative activities. While there were no differences between the two groups studied before they started their activities, following the intense mindfulness exercises, the group doing the meditation exercises exhibited a down-regulation of genes that have been implicated in inflammation. This means that the rate of gene expression was decreased in these genes, which could result in reduced inflammation. Genes do not direct all of an organism's functions; rather they interact and respond to the environment. This could mean that by using mindfulness practices, the negative effects we discussed in terms of stress and psychoneuroimmunology may be combated (see Chapter 4). This type of research is beginning to uncover the precise ways mind–body approaches such as mindfulness and meditation work, and may act as scientific verification of some of the reported benefits of such techniques. In turn this type of evidence demonstrates the processes that occur when engaging in such activities and will therefore make it more possible for healthcare providers to offer mind–body approaches to people with conditions such as CFS/ME.

Summary and conclusion

Overall the future looks very promising indeed for people with conditions such as CFS/ME. There have been concerted efforts within the research community to increase communication, collaboration and the amount of research into the condition. Already there have been exciting developments in terms of the resources being generated for researchers to use, such as the UK ME/CFS Biobank. Funders are becoming increasingly interested in CFS/ME and more and more researchers are being attracted to working in the area. There is of course a great deal more work to do, but if you take nothing else from this book, know that there are many dedicated people working to provide greater understanding, more treatment options and further guidance on how you can recover from CFS/ME.

Useful addresses

CFS/ME charities

Action for ME
PO Box 2778
Bristol BS1 9DJ
Tel.: 0845 123 2380 (lo-call);
0117 927 9551 (9 a.m. to 5 p.m., Monday to Friday)
Website: www.actionforme.org.uk

CFIDS Association of America
PO Box 220398
Charlotte, NC 28222-0398
Tel.: 00 1 704 365 2343
Website: http://solvecfs.org

ME Association
7 Apollo Office Court
Radclive Road
Gawcott
Buckingham MK18 4DF
Tel.: 01280 818964 (9.30 a.m. to 3.30 p.m.)
Website: www.meassociation.org.uk

Complementary and alternative treatments

British Acupuncture Council
63 Jeddo Road
London W12 9HQ
Tel.: 020 8735 0400
Fax: 020 8735 0404
Website: www.acupuncture.org.uk

British Council for Yoga Therapy
Website: www.bcyt.co.uk

Complementary and Natural Healthcare Council
83 Victoria Street
London SW1H 0HW
Tel.: 020 3178 2199 (9.30 a.m. to 5.30 p.m., Monday to Friday)
Website: www.chnc.org.uk

General Hypnotherapy Standards Council (GHSC) and
General Hypnotherapy Register (GHR)
PO Box 204
Lymington
Hants SO41 6WP
Website: www.general-hypnotherapy-register.com

Hypnotherapy Association UK
14 Crown Street
Chorley
Lancashire PR6 1DX
Tel.: 01257 262124
Website: www.thehypnotherapyassociation.co.uk

National Hypnotherapy Society
PO Box 131
Arundel
West Sussex BN18 8BR
Tel.: 0870 850 3387
Website: www.nationalhypnotherapysociety.org

Yoga Alliance
1701 Clarendon Boulevard, Suite 100
Arlington, VA 22209
Tel.: 00 1 888 921 9642 or 00 1 571 482 3355 (9 a.m. to 6 p.m., USA Eastern
Standard Time)
Website: www.yogaalliance.org

Other

For information on the 'Any Other Provider' scheme visit:
www.nhs.uk/choiceinthenhs/yourchoices/any-qualified-provider/Pages/
aqp.aspx

National Institute for Health and Care Excellence (NICE)
Guidelines for CFS may be accessed at
http://guidance.nice.org.uk/CG53

Selected references

Carruthers, B. M., Jain, A. K., de Meirleir, K. L., Peterson, D. L., Klimas, N. G. et al. (2003). 'Myalgic Encephalomyelitis/Chronic Fatigue Syndrome: Clinical Working Case Definition, Diagnostic and Treatment Protocols'. *Journal of Chronic Fatigue Syndrome*, 11(1), 7–36.

Dancey, C. P. and Friend, J. (2008). 'Symptoms, Impairment and Illness Intrusiveness – Their Relationship with Depression in Women with CFS/ME'. *Psychology and Health*, 23(8), 983–99.

Devasahayam, A., Lawn, T., Murphy, M. and White, P. D. (2012). 'Alternative Diagnoses to Chronic Fatigue Syndrome in Referrals to a Specialist Service: Service Evaluation Survey'. *JRSM Short Reports*, 3(1).

Edmonds, M., McGuire, H. and Price, J. (2004). 'Exercise Therapy for Chronic Fatigue Syndrome'. *The Cochrane Database of Systematic Reviews*, 3, 1–25.

Engel, G. L. (1977). 'The Need for a New Medical Model: A Challenge for Biomedicine'. *Science*, 196(4286), 129–36.

Fukuda, K., Straus, S. E., Hickie, I., Sharpe, M. C., Dobbins, J. G. and Komaroff, A. (1994). 'The Chronic Fatigue Syndrome: A Comprehensive Approach to its Definition and Study'. *Annals of Internal Medicine*, 121, 953–9.

Glaser, R. (2005). 'Stress-Associated Immune Dysregulation and its Importance for Human Health: A Personal History of Psychoneuroimmunology'. *Brain, Behavior, and Immunity*, 19(1), 3–11.

Harvey, S. B., Wadsworth, M., Wessely, S. and Hotopf, M. (2008). 'Etiology of Chronic Fatigue Syndrome: Testing Popular Hypotheses Using a National Birth Cohort Study'. *Psychosomatic Medicine*, 70, 488–95.

Hatcher, S. and House, A. (2003). 'Life Events, Difficulties and Dilemmas in the Onset of Chronic Fatigue Syndrome: A Case-Control Study'. *Psychological Medicine*, 33(7), 1185–92.

Holmes, G. P., Kaplan, J. E., Gantz, N. M., Komaroff, A. L., Schonberger, L. B., Straus, S. E., . . . Schooley, R. T. (1988). 'Chronic Fatigue Syndrome: A Working Case Definition'. *Annals of Internal Medicine*, 108(3), 387–9.

Jason, L., Jessen, T., Porter, N., Boulton, A. and Gloria-Njoku, M. (2009). 'Examining Types of Fatigue Among Individuals with ME/CFS'. *Disability Studies Quarterly*, 29(3).

Kiecolt-Glaser, J. K. and Glaser, R. (1989). 'Psychoneuro-Immunology: Past, Present and Future'. *Health Psychology*, 8, 677–82.

Krupp, L. B., Jandorf, L., Coyle, P. K. and Mendelson, W. B. (1993). 'Sleep Disturbance in Chronic Fatigue Syndrome'. *Journal of Psychosomatic Research*, 37(4), 325–31.

Levine, P. H., Jacobson, S., Pocinki, A. G., Cheney, P., Peterson, D. et al. (1992). 'Clinical, Epidemiologic, and Virologic Studies in Four Clusters of the Chronic Fatigue Syndrome'. *Archives of Internal Medicine*, 152(8), 1611–6.

McEvedy, C. P. and Beard, A. (1970). 'Royal Free Epidemic of 1955: A Reconsideration'. *British Medical Journal*, 1(5687), 7–11.

Maes, M. and Twisk, F. N. M. (2010). 'Chronic Fatigue Syndrome: Harvey and Wessely's (Bio)psychosocial Model Versus a Bio(Psychosocial) Model Based on Inflammatory and Oxidative and Nitrosative Stress Pathways'. *BMC Medicine*, 8(35), 35–47.

Myhill, S., Booth, N. E. and McLaren-Howard, J. (2009). 'Chronic Fatigue Syndrome and Mitochondrial Dysfunction'. *International Journal of Clinical and Experimental Medicine*, 2(1), 1–16.

Newton, J., Mabillard, H., Scott, A., Hoad, A. and Spickett, G. (2010). 'The Newcastle NHS Chronic Fatigue Syndrome Service: Not all Fatigue is the Same'. *The Journal of the Royal College of Physicians of Edinburgh*, 40(4), 304–7.

Price, J. R., Mitchell, E., Tidy, E. and Hunot, V. (2008). 'Cognitive Behaviour Therapy for Chronic Fatigue Syndrome in Adults'. *Cochrane Database of Systematic Reviews*, (Issue 3).

Roberts, A. D. L., Wessely, S., Chalder, T., Papadopoulos, A. and Cleare, A. J. (2004). 'Salivary Cortisol Response to Awakening in Chronic Fatigue Syndrome'. *British Journal of Psychiatry*, 184(2), 136–41.

Snell, C. R., Stevens, S. R., Davenport, T. E. and Van Ness, J. M. (2013). 'Discriminative Validity of Metabolic and Workload Measurements for Identifying People with Chronic Fatigue Syndrome'. *Physical Therapy*, 93(11), 1484–92.

Taylor, R. R. and Kielhofner, G. W. (2005). 'Work-related Impairment and Employment-Focused Rehabilitation Options for Individuals with Chronic Fatigue Syndrome: A Review'. *Journal of Mental Health*, 14(3), 253–67.

Van Houdenhove, B., Neerinckx, E., Onghena, P., Lysens, R. and Vertommen, H. (2001). 'Premorbid "overactive" Lifestyle in Chronic Fatigue Syndrome and Fibromyalgia: An Etiological Factor or Proof of Good Citizenship?' *Journal of Psychosomatic Research*, 51(4), 571–6.

Ware, N. C. (1992). 'Suffering and the Social Construction of Illness: The Delegitimation of Illness Experience in Chronic Fatigue Syndrome'. *Medical Anthropology Quarterly*, 6, 347–61.

Index